FOOD FOR PREGNANCY:

3 Manuscripts in 1

MIA ANGELS

FOOD FOR PREGNANCY VOLUME 1

*The Moms Guide to Understanding the Best Supplements
and Nutrients for A Healthy Growing Baby*

INTRODUCTION

Pregnancy is one of the most beautiful stages in a woman's life. Most of the time, you are not told about what you will need to live through during your pregnancy. You are also not warned about the many changes that you will need to make to your lifestyle. Truth be told, pregnancy is not a fairytale, and it is important that you are prepared for a few things. There are some that you will be aware about, but there are some things that are often concealed from you, and it is important that you know what these things are.

Pregnancy will change the way you lead your life, and it will change you forever. You will need to change the way you eat, and remember that you are eating for two people. Now when most women hear this, they believe that they need to double their food intake. What they do not realize is that they need to focus on what they are eating and not how much food they are eating. You should ensure that you consume food that is nutritious and healthy for you and your baby.

If you have recently found out that you are pregnant, you will have been given enough advice on what food you should eat and what you shouldn't. The amount of information thrown at you may have overwhelmed you. This book will put you at ease. You will learn everything you need to know about nutrition and the type of food you should eat.

Over the course of the book, you will learn more about why it is important for you to eat well, and the different nutrients you will need to consume regularly. You will also gather information on the different types of food you are allowed to eat and those that you must avoid. Remember that you should avoid some foods at all costs to keep your baby safe. You will also be given a few tips that will help you maintain your weight and obtain the required nutrition. It is important for you to remember that you will be consuming food for two people, and you should increase your intake of some nutrients to promote your health and your baby's health.

Thank you for purchasing the book. I hope the information in the book will help you learn more about how to stay healthy during your pregnancy.

Chapter One

IMPORTANCE OF FOOD DURING PREGNANCY

*I*t is always important to consider what type of food you are eating during your pregnancy, and not look at the quantity. Studies show that women only need to consume 450 extra calories during their pregnancy, and this is only when the baby starts to grow quickly. You can easily consume these extra calories by consuming a bowl of cereal with full-fat milk. Even if you increase your food intake, you should ensure that you consume only nutritious food since this will help with the development and growth of your baby.

Eating Well When You're Pregnant

Most women are surprised to note that they have gained 35 pounds during their pregnancy, especially when a baby weighs only a quarter of that. The pounds that you gain will add up in the following manner, but this will vary from one woman to another.

- 7.5 pounds: The weight of your baby

- 7 pounds: The stored fat, protein and other macro and micro nutrients
- 4 pounds: The extra blood
- 4 pounds: The extra fluids in the body
- 2 pounds: The large breasts
- 2 pounds: Your uterus enlarging
- 2 pounds: The amniotic fluid that surrounds your baby
- 1.5 pounds: The placenta in the womb

It is true that the pattern of weight gain will vary from one woman to another during their pregnancy. There are some women who will gain less weight if they were already heavy before they were pregnant, while there are others who will weigh a lot more if they have triplets or twins. You may also gain very little weight if you were underweight before your pregnancy. It is okay to gain weight, but it is important to know why you have gained that weight. The main source of nourishment for your baby is the food that you consume during your pregnancy. It was only recently that people began to understand that there is a very strong link between the food that you consume and the health of your baby. It is for this reason that doctors say that you should never drink alcohol, even if it is a small amount, during your pregnancy.

It is important for you to remember that the extra food that you consume should not only be calories. The food should be nutritious. For instance, calcium will help to keep your bones and teeth strong, and when you consume extra calcium you will be strengthening your baby's bones. The same can be said about all the food that you eat.

Nutrition for Expectant Moms
A balanced diet will include carbohydrates, proteins, vita-

mins, fats, minerals and at least two liters of water. You can use the guidelines provided by the US government to determine the number of servings of food that you should consume every day. It is always a good idea to consume different types of food since that will help you stay healthy.

Every packet of food that you purchase will have a food label that will tell you about the different types of nutrients in that food. The recommended daily allowance or RDA that is present on the food label will tell you what quantity of each nutrient you should consume every day. The RDA for most nutrients is usually high when you are pregnant.

Let us look at some nutrients that you should consume, and the food that contain those nutrients:

- Protein: This nutrient is essential for blood production and cell growth. The best sources of food for this nutrient are poultry, beans, egg whites, peanut butter, lean meat, fish and tofu.
- Carbohydrates: This nutrient is essential for the production of energy. The best sources of food for this nutrient are cereals, potatoes, rice, breads, fruit, vegetables and pasta.
- Calcium: This nutrient is essential to maintain the strength of teeth and bones, for muscle contraction and nerve function. The best sources of food for this nutrient are cheese, milk, sardines, salmon, yogurt and spinach.
- Iron: This nutrient is essential for the production of red blood cells to prevent anemia. The best sources of food for this nutrient are spinach, lean red meat, whole-grain and iron-fortified cereals and breads.
- Vitamin A: This nutrient is essential to maintain good eyesight, aid in the growth of bones and to

maintain healthy skin. The best sources of food for
this nutrient are dark leafy greens, carrots and
sweet potatoes.

- Vitamin C: This nutrient is essential to maintain
healthy teeth and gums. It also improves the body's
ability to absorb iron. The best sources of food for
this nutrient are broccoli, citrus fruit, fortified
juices and tomatoes.
- Vitamin B6: This nutrient improves the body's
ability to effectively use carbohydrates, fats and
protein. The best sources of food for this nutrient
are whole-grain cereals, pork, banana and ham.
- Vitamin B12: This nutrient is used to maintain and
improve the functioning of the nervous system.
The best sources of food for this nutrient are milk,
poultry, fish and meat.
- Vitamin D: This nutrient helps to improve the
body's ability to absorb calcium. The best sources
of food for this nutrient are dairy products, breads,
cereals and fortified milk.
- Folic Acid: The benefits of this nutrient have been
discussed in detail in the next chapter. The best
sources of food for this nutrient are dark yellow
fruit, beans, nuts, green leafy vegetables and peas.
- Fat: This nutrient is stored as energy in the body.
The sources of food for this nutrient are nuts,
meat, peanut butter, whole-milk products,
vegetable oils and margarine.

Every scientist is aware that your baby's health is dependent on the food that you consume. You should take care of
your diet even before you are pregnant. For instance, studies
show that folic acid is one of the only nutrients that can help
to reduce the risk of developing neural tube defects during

the early development stages of the fetus. It is for this reason that it is important that you consume this mineral in large quantities before your pregnancy and during the first few weeks of your pregnancy.

Doctors always suggest that women should take supplements for folic acids during their pregnancy, especially for the first four weeks. If you are considering pregnancy, you should speak to your doctor about your intake of folic acid. Another important nutrient that you should consider is calcium. This mineral is essential for the development and growth of your baby. Since your baby will absorb the calcium from the food that you contain, you should increase your intake to prevent any loss of calcium from your bones. Your doctor will also give you some prenatal vitamins that will have more folic acid and calcium.

The best sources of calcium are dairy products and milk. If you are lactose intolerant or are nauseous when you drink milk or consume dairy products, you can request your doctor to prescribe some calcium supplements. You are lactose intolerant if you develop gas, have bloating around your stomach and have diarrhea when you eat milk products or drink milk. You can either use lactose-free milk products or take a lactase capsule to help you digest the lactose. Other foods that are rich in calcium are salmon with bones, sardines, broccoli, tofu, calcium-fortified juices and spinach.

It is recommended that you do not begin a vegan diet during your pregnancy. If you were always a vegetarian or a vegan, you can continue this diet during your pregnancy, but you will need to be careful about the food that you eat. It will be difficult to obtain the right nutrition when you do not consume chicken, fish, eggs, milk and cheese. You will need to take protein supplements and Vitamin D and Vitamin B12 supplements.

You should consult a physician and a nutritionist during

your pregnancy to ensure that you and your baby receive the required nutrition.

Food Cravings During Pregnancy

You probably know many women who have had cravings during their pregnancy, and you may have had some cravings yourself. There are some theories that state that a woman's craving for a specific type of food during pregnancy will indicate that the woman's body lacks the nutrients present in that food. This is definitely not a correct assumption, and doctors and researchers are still unsure why women have these cravings.

During their pregnancy, some women crave fruit, comfort food like cereals, mashed potatoes and toasted bread, chocolates and spicy food. Some women also crave cornstarch, clay and other non-food items, and this type of eating is called pica. If you consume things that are not food, you will endanger yourself and your baby. If you find yourself having some non-food cravings, you should consult your doctor immediately.

It is okay to give into your cravings if you ensure that you consume nutritious food in your other meals. You will find yourself craving for different types of food only during the first few months of your pregnancy.

Food and Drinks to Avoid While Pregnant

You should never consume alcohol during your pregnancy because it is not safe for you or your baby. You should also check with your doctor before you consume any herbal products or take any vitamin supplements since they can harm the development and growth of the fetus. There are some doctors who say that you can consume two cups of coffee, soda or tea every day since this amount of caffeine will not harm you or your baby. That said, it is wise to avoid caffeine altogether if you can since caffeine can lead to numerous problems and miscarriage. Try to switch to decaffeinated products or limit your intake of caffeine. We will look at some of the different foods that you should avoid in the last chapter of the book.

Managing Some Common Problems

- *Constipation*

Pregnant women often have constipation because of the iron that is present in the prenatal vitamins. There are numerous other factors that can cause constipation too. It is for this reason that you should eat more fiber during your pregnancy. Try to consume at least thirty grams of fiber every day. The best sources for fiber are cereals, whole-grain breads, muffins, fruit and vegetables.

There are some people who use substitutes in the form of drinks or tablets, but it is important that you check with your doctor before you consume these products. You should avoid using laxatives unless your doctor specifically asks you to consume them. You should also avoid drinking castor oil since it will affect your body's ability to absorb the required vitamins and minerals from the food you consume.

If you have constipation regularly, you should ask your doctor for a stool softener. You should ensure that you drink a lot of water and increase your intake of fiber. If you do not do this, you will make the constipation worse. If you have the energy, you should try to exercise since this helps to avoid constipation. Drink enough water during the day. Always drink two glasses of water after your meal to make it easier for you to move the food through the digestive system. You can also consume broth, soups or tea.

- **Gas**

Food like spinach, broccoli, fried foods and cauliflower can give some women gas or heartburn during their pregnancy. If you feel that this happens to you, you should consume a diet where you consume substitutes for these foods. You should also try to avoid carbonated drinks since they can cause heartburn and gas.

- **Nausea**

Most women are nauseated during the first trimester. So, instead of avoiding food, you should try to consume small portions of food that is bland, like crackers or toast. You can also consume food that is made with ginger. Let us look at a few tips that will help you combat nausea.

1. Never take your prenatal vitamins on an empty stomach. It is recommended that you consume these vitamins before you go to bed if you have eaten a snack.
2. Try to consume a small snack whenever you wake up in the morning to use the washroom.
3. Try to suck on hard candy.

Chapter Two

IMPORTANT NUTRIENTS

*N*ow that you know why it is important to focus on the type of food you are eating, let us look at some of the macronutrients and micronutrients that you should consume during your pregnancy.

Macronutrients

- *Energy*

The amount of energy you consume will determine the amount of weight you gain during your pregnancy. It is important to remember that you will need to eat the required amount of energy during your pregnancy to ensure that you supply your body with the usual amount and also support the growth and development of the fetus. The extra energy that you consume will help in the growth and development of existing tissue and new tissue. You will not find that you need more energy during the first trimester of your pregnancy. It is only from the second trimester that you will need more energy. The growth of the tissue in the mother and the fetus is more from the second trimester. That said, the energy that a pregnant woman needs during her pregnancy is dependent on many other factors like the body mass index (BMI) before pregnancy, the metabolic rate and the physical activity levels. Therefore, you should tailor your need for energy depending on your body.

The global estimate suggests that pregnant women need to consume at least 9260 kJ of energy per day. You must ensure that you provide your body with the required amount of energy to reduce the risk of miscarriages, premature birth and stillbirth. When you provide your body with less energy, your weight will automatically reduce. There is, however, very little research to determine whether the consumption of energy can be restricted.

A study was conducted on 384 subjects, and an analysis was made based on three trials. This study reported that women who gained too much weight during pregnancy or were overweight before pregnancy can reduce their consumption of energy to obtain their ideal gestational weight. Two of these trials, however, reported that any reduction in the consumption of energy could have adverse effects on the baby's birth weight. It is important to prevent maternal obesity, but it is also important to reduce the risk of any complications during birth. Given that there is very little evidence, it is advised that pregnant women do not reduce the consumption of energy.

- ### *Protein*

Protein is a macronutrient that is required for both structural and functional biological roles. The primary source of protein across the globe is from plant-based foods like grains, nuts and legumes, followed by animal-based foods and dairy.

There are some alternative sources for protein like bacteria, fungi and algae. These are known as micro proteins. The quality of protein is determined based on its capacity to meet the requirement of amino acids and nitrogen that are necessary for maintenance, growth and repair and its digestibility. Animal protein is termed as a complete protein since it provides the required quantity of nitrogen and indispensable amino acids. The plant-based proteins are incomplete proteins since they will be deficient in at least one protein like threonine or lysine.

Based on the current recommendations by the US Government, the consumption of at least 16.1% protein of the total energy is adequate for pregnant women. There will be some adjustments that your body makes in the protein metabolism during the first few weeks of pregnancy. This is done to maintain homeostasis in the mother's body while accommodating the needs and demands of the fetus. Studies show that protein is synthesized in large quantities from the second trimester to cater to the fetus' needs. If you are well nourished, these changes will help to conserve nitrogen and protein, and also promote the accumulation of protein to ensure that the fetus obtains the required nutrition.

• *Fiber, Glycemic Index and Glycemic Load*

You can obtain carbohydrates from numerous sources, and each of these foods has a different digestion rate. Therefore, the effect of these foods will affect the insulin levels and the blood glucose levels differently. The glycemic index for each source will quantify your body's response that is induced by the carbohydrates. Foods like white bread, potatoes and rice have a high glycemic index, and they cause a sharp increase in the blood glucose levels when consumed. The levels also decline rapidly once the food has been digested.

Foods like dairy products and fruit have a low glycemic index, and the carbohydrates in these foods are digested slowly. This results in a low response to glucose. The glycemic load will look at both the quantity of carbohydrates and the glycemic index of the food. You can calculate the glycemic load in food by multiplying the carbohydrate content with the glycemic index.

The dietary fiber is the plant-based carbohydrate that we consume. These carbohydrates cannot be digested by the human digestive system. Dietary fiber includes starch resistant fiber that is obtained from cooked rice and potato, and soluble fiber, which is obtained from vegetables, fruit and legumes. Doctors and researchers advise women to consume food with a low glycemic index and glycemic load, and food that is rich in fiber to modulate and maintain the blood glucose levels, reduce constipation and also reduce the cholesterol levels in blood.

- **Fatty Acids**

Down of the essential fatty acids are the short-chain fatty acids including alpha-linoleic and linoleic acids, and the long-chain derivatives including Docosahexaenoic acid (DHA), Eicosapentaenoic acid (EPA) and Arachidonic acid (AA). These fatty acids are required for the formation of tissues and are used to build the cell membranes. Some foods that are rich in these fatty acids include oily fish like salmon and mackerel and some fish oil supplements. The concentration of these fats decreases in the body during pregnancy by at least 40%. Therefore, it is important that a woman increase her intake of fatty acids, especially the long-chain fatty acids during pregnancy. This is the only way that the mother can meet the dietary requirements of her body and the fetus. DHA can help to develop the retina and brain in the fetus.

EPA can help to reduce the production of thromboxane A2. If you are unable to consume the required quantity of Vitamin D through your diet, you should ask your doctor to suggest some supplements.

Micronutrients in Pregnancy

- *Folate*

Folate is present in yeast extract, citrus fruit like oranges and leafy green vegetables. It is a water-soluble vitamin. There are some breakfast cereals and bread that are fortified with folic acid, which is the more stable and synthetic form of folate. This vitamin acts as a coenzyme during the methylation cycles in the body, and helps to transfer carbon through the body. It is integral for the synthesis of neurotransmitters and DNA. This vitamin is also used in the synthesis of proteins, multiplication of cells and the metabolism of amino acids. This makes it important for pregnant women to increase their intake of folate during the first few weeks of pregnancy since the fetus will grow rapidly because of cell division and growth of tissues. Deficiency of folate will result in the accumulation of homocysteine. This will increase the risk of preeclampsia and anomalies or abnormalities in the fetus.

It is important to consume folic acid during the first few weeks of pregnancy to reduce the risk of developing neural tube defects. The neural tube is developed in the first few weeks of pregnancy, and it is important to take folic acid supplements to aid in the growth of the tube.

- *Vitamin A*

Vitamin A can be derived from provitamin carotenoids and preformed retinoids. Retinoids, like retinoic acid and retinal acid, can be obtained from different animal sources including fish liver oil, liver, dairy and eggs. Carotenoids like beta-carotene can be obtained from numerous plants like yellow or dark vegetables like sweet potatoes, carrots and kale. These compounds are converted into Vitamin A by the body, and stored in the liver. Some physiological functions of Vitamin A are bone metabolism, growth, gene transcription and immune function. This vitamin enhances the antioxidant activities in the body. Women are advised to consume more vitamin A during pregnancy since this vitamin will be used to support the growth of the fetus and maintain the tissues. If you are unable to obtain the required intake of Vitamin A, you can consume supplements. The effects of vitamin A on the body during pregnancy vary, and further research needs to be conducted to understand this better. It is, however, important that women monitor the levels of Vitamin A in their body to ensure that the vitamin is not being accumulated in the liver leading to toxicity.

- ***Vitamin B_1 (Thiamine), Vitamin B_3 (Niacin), Vitamin B_6 (Pyridoxine), Vitamin B_2 (Riboflavin), and Vitamin B_{12} (Cyanocobalamin)***

Vitamin B is a complex vitamin, and it includes B_1 (Thiamine), B_3 (Niacin), B_6 (Pyridoxine), B_2 (Riboflavin), and B_{12} (Cyanocobalamin). These vitamins are water-soluble and are used by the body for the production of energy in cells. It is also required for the metabolism of fats, carbohydrates and protein. These vitamins also act as coenzymes, and is used in numerous metabolic pathways for the formation of blood cells and also in the generation of energy. Vitamin B12 works with Folate to generate methionine from homocysteine. This process is required for the methylation of neurotransmitters, phospholipids, proteins, DNA and RNA. A deficiency in these vitamins will negatively impact the growth of cells and the growth of nerve tissues. Women are advised to take prenatal vitamins during pregnancy, and these vitamins contain Vitamin B.

Vitamin B-complex can be found in large quantities in fortified cereals, leafy green vegetables, legumes and animal products including dairy products, fish, poultry and meat. Pregnant women are required to increase their intake of vitamin B since there is an increase in the protein and energy required by the body.

- ### *Vitamin C and E*

Vitamin E and Vitamin C are fat-soluble and water-soluble vitamins. Vitamin E is a group of eight compounds that are obtained from plants, of which four compounds are toco-tienols, namely alpha, beta, gamma and delta, and four toco-pherols, namely alpha, beta, gamma and delta. The alpha-tocopherol is a biologically active compound. Vitamin C can be found in a variety of fruit and vegetables like citrus fruit, broccoli, tomatoes and guava. Vitamin E can be found in vegetable oils, wheat germ oil, some leafy vegetables and nuts. Vitamins C and E increase the formation of radicals in the body, which help to reduce oxidative stress. These vitamins also improve the immune system. Vitamin C also increases the synthesis of collagen. This compound is one of the primary components of connective tissues, and enhances the body's ability to absorb iron, thereby reducing iron deficiency and preventing megaloblastic anemia.

During pregnancy, the body transports the vitamin C consumed into the placenta. This reduces the amount of

Vitamin C in the mother's body thereby increasing the daily intake to 85 milligrams a day.

- ***Vitamin D***

Vitamin D is an essential nutrient required to maintain the integrity of bones and also maintain calcium homeostasis in the body. Vitamin D is also required for the performance of some extra skeletal functions including its role in reducing inflammation, improving the function of the immune system, angiogenesis and the metabolism of glucose. It is also used in the regulation of gene expression and transcription. The body absorbs Vitamin D when it is exposed to the sun. You can also obtain Vitamin D from few foods like fortified dairy products and oily fish. If you do not meet the required intake of Vitamin D, you can take some supplements in the form of ergocalciferol (vitamin D2) and cholecalciferol (vitamin D3).

When Vitamin D is synthesized or ingested, it is first broken down in the liver to form the Vitamin hydroxyvitamin D (25(OH) D). This form of the vitamin is what can be circulated. The quantity of this form of the vitamin in the body is used to determine if there is a deficiency or not. Vitamin D is also broken down in the kidneys to create the active form of the vitamin, 1,25-dihydroxyvitamin D (1,25(OH) 2D3).

The deficiency of Vitamin D can be attributed to pigmented skin, lack of exposure to sunlight because of a sedentary lifestyle, the use of protective clothing or sunscreen and a low intake of fortified foods. It is important to control your intake of Vitamin D and also to prevent a deficiency especially during pregnancy.

- ***Calcium***

Calcium is one of the most essential nutrients to

strengthen bones. It is also an important component that is found in the membranes around the cells. This mineral is used in numerous biological processes including muscle contractions, hormone homeostasis, signal transduction and enzyme homeostasis. It is also important to improve the function of neurons. Some of the best sources of calcium are dairy products and milk, but this mineral can also be obtained from fortified foods like dairy alternatives and flour, leafy green vegetables and nuts.

During pregnancy, the mother's body will automatically transfer the calcium from the placenta into the fetus. It is for this reason that the mother's need for calcium increases, especially during the third trimester. Calcium is used efficiently during pregnancy because of the changes made to the mother's physiology. During pregnancy, a woman's body will absorb more calcium because of the hormonal changes in the body. The kidneys will also retain calcium in their tubules during pregnancy. A woman can meet the required intake of calcium through her diet alone, but supplements can be taken to ensure that there is a balance in the calcium levels in the woman's body.

Calcium deficiency can lead to paresthesia, tetanus, tremors, muscle cramps and osteopenia. It can also lead to delayed growth in the fetus, poor mineralization in the bones and LBW. Studies show that women who consume very little calcium may develop hypertensive disorders during pregnancy.

- *Iodine*

Iron is one of the many nutrients that aids in regulating metabolism, growth and development through the synthesis of the triiodothyronine (T3) and thyroxine (T4) hormones. This nutrient is obtained from fortified salt, but can also be sourced from various seafood and kelp. Iodine can also be obtained from plant and dairy products that have been sourced from iodine-fortified animal feed or sowed in iodine-rich soil. The hormonal alterations and metabolic demands during pregnancy increase the need for iodine. The demands increase because the production of the thyroid hormone during the first trimester increases by 50% and the excretion of iodine also increases by 50%. It is only later during the gestation period that the iodine is passed through the placenta to the fetus.

The thyroid hormones in the mother and the fetus regulate some of the key development processes. The hormones regulate the development of the nervous system in the fetus, and also aid in the formation of the myelination and synapses, and the growth of the nerve cells. You will only need to consume small quantities of iodine to prevent deficiency. However, iodine deficiency disorders are the main reason behind cognitive impairments in the fetus. Other consequences of iodine deficiencies are lower Intelligent Quotient (IQ) in children, stillbirth, miscarriage and fetal goiter.

- **Iron**

Iron is essential for the synthesis of myoglobin and hemoglobin in the blood. It is a vital nutrient used for numerous cellular functions including respiration, oxygen transport, Gene regulation, growth and the functioning of those enzymes that are made up of iron. It is for this reason that it is necessary that the right quantity of iron is stored in the body to ensure homeostasis. Having said that, iron deficiency is one of the most common deficiencies across the world. Pregnant women have low iron content in their body because they do not consume the right food to improve the body's ability to absorb iron. They may also have iron deficiency if they are affected by any parasites. It is for this reason that it is important to increase your intake of plant-based foods like green leafy vegetables. These vegetables contain non-heam iron used in different bodily functions. That said, the body absorbs the heam iron from animal meat and fish easily, and it is because of this that these products are the main source of iron for mammals.

During pregnancy, the need for iron increases to 7.5 milligrams a day, although it is hard to determine the amount required during the third trimester. Iron is needed to fulfill the needs of the fetus, for the expansion of the erythrocyte mass in the mother and to compensate for the loss of iron. Since the iron required during pregnancy increases during pregnancy, the chances of developing an iron deficiency also increase. A study conducted by WHO concluded that close to 38.2% pregnant women have an iron deficiency and are anemic.

Anemia and iron deficiency are known to increase the risk of premature birth, SGA or LBW infants, lower immunity against diseases and infection, impaired bodily functions in the mother and abnormal development of cognitive function and psychomotor development in the fetus.

- *Zinc*

Zinc is one of the most important nutrients that one should consume because it contains over 200 enzymes and is a structural component in numerous hormones, proteins and nucleotides. This mineral has the most important biochemical functions since it aids in the synthesis of proteins and also helps to break down nucleic acids in the human body. This mineral also aids in gene expression, cellular division, wound healing, immune and neurological function, antioxidant defenses and vision.

Zinc can be found in different types of food, but large quantities of this mineral are found in seafood, nuts, milk and meat. Diets that are rich in fiber will reduce the quantity of zinc found in the body. The amount of zinc present in the body can be measured by checking the levels of zinc in the plasma or serum. The values will vary depending on the sex, age, physiological factors like infection or stress and the time of day. Due to this it becomes difficult for people to accurately determine whether they are deficient. It is, however, estimated that close to 82 percent of pregnant women are deficient in zinc. Doctors recommend that pregnant women consume at least fifteen milligrams of zinc from the second trimester.

Studies show that close to half a million child and maternal deaths a year occur due to deficiency in zinc, and this is especially true for developing countries. Deficiency in zinc has been associated with prolonged labor, intrauterine growth retardation, pregnancy-induced hypertension, LBW, impaired immunity and pre-term and post-term births. If your body has trouble with absorbing zinc, it can lead to a miscarriage or congenital malfunctions.

Two separate studies were conducted to understand the effects of zinc during pregnancy. These studies reported that the use of zinc supplements during pregnancy helped to reduce the risk of premature birth by at least fourteen percent. That said, there was no effect of these supplements on the neonatal mortality, birth weight and hypertensive disorders. Doctors believe that zinc helps to reduce the risk of premature birth by reducing the risk of infections during pregnancy.

Chapter Three

HEALTHY FOODS EQUALS HEALTHY BABY

*a*s mentioned earlier, it is important to ensure that you maintain your health during pregnancy. It is during this time that you will need to provide your body with additional vitamins, minerals and nutrients. As mentioned earlier, you will need to increase your intake of calories by 450, but will also need to focus on the nutrition. If you consume food that is not nutritious, it will impact the development of the baby. Excess weight gain and poor eating habits can increase the risk of complications during birth and gestational diabetes. In simple terms, if you choose to consume nutritious food, you can ensure the health of your baby and yourself. It will also make it very easy for you to lose all the weight you put on during pregnancy once you give birth. This chapter lists some of the best foods that you should consume during your pregnancy.

Dairy Products

It is important for you to increase your intake of calcium and protein during pregnancy to ensure that you meet the needs of your baby. There are two high-quality proteins that are found in dairy products – whey and casein. Dairy is also one of the best sources of calcium, and it provides large quantities of magnesium, Vitamin B, zinc and phosphorous. Doctors advise pregnant women to consume yogurt, especially Greek yogurt since that contains more protein and calcium when compared to other dairy products. There are some types of yogurt that also contain probiotic bacteria that aid in digestion. If you are lactose intolerant, you may be able to tolerate probiotic yogurt. You can also take some probiotic supplements to reduce the risk of any complications that may arise during pregnancy like vaginal infections, gestational diabetes, preeclampsia and allergies.

Legumes

Legumes are a group of food that includes peas, lentils, chickpeas, peanuts, beans and soybeans. Legumes are rich in protein, folate, calcium and iron, and they are the best source of fiber. Your body needs each of these nutrients in large quantities during pregnancy. Folate is an essential vitamin that helps to maintain the health of both the fetus and the mother. Unfortunately, most women do not consume the required quantity of folate during their pregnancy, which can lead to low birth weight and neural tube defects. It is for this reason that you should increase your intake of folate during the first trimester. Insufficient folate can also impact your child's immune system, which can render him or her defenseless to some diseases and infections. Legumes are rich in folate, and one serving of lentils provides at least ninety percent of the required intake of folate.

Sweet Potatoes

Sweet potatoes are rich in a plant compound called beta-carotene. This compound helps to convert the vitamin A in the human body into a useable form. This vitamin aids in the development and growth of the tissues and cells in the fetus, and is extremely important for the development of the fetus. Doctors recommend that pregnant women should increase their intake of Vitamin A by at least 40 percent. That said, they are also advised to reduce their intake of Vitamin A from animal-based sources since this can lead to toxicity in the body. Sweet potatoes are rich in beta-carotene, and one cup of cooked sweet potato a day is enough to fulfill the daily requirement of beat-carotene. Sweet potatoes also contain fiber. This nutrient will reduce the spikes in blood sugar, improve digestion, improve mobility and satiate your hunger.

Salmon

Salmon is one of the best sources of omega-3 fatty acids, and most people, especially pregnant women, do not consume the required amount of omega-3 fatty acids through their diet. The long chain Omega-3 fatty acids like EPA and DHA are essential during pregnancy, and these acids are found in large quantities in seafood. They help in the growth and development of your fetus's eyes and brain. That said, women are advised to limit their intake of seafood to twice a week or lesser depending on the Mercury content in the fish. Since Mercury is a fatal compound, most women avoid fish altogether because they worry about their baby. This limits their intake of Omega-3 fatty acids. Studies show that Willem who consume at least two meals of low-mercury and fatty-fish consume the required amount of omega-3 fatty acids. This helps to increase the levels of EPA and DHA in the blood. Salmon is one of the very few natural sources of Vitamin D, and this is a vitamin that is lacking in most people's diet. This vitamin endures the health of your bones, improves the function of the immune system and aids numerous processes that take place in the human body.

Eggs

Eggs are the best food to consume since they contain every nutrient that your body needs. One large egg is rich is high-quality fat and protein, and adds 77 calories to your diet. This food is also rich in numerous vitamins and minerals. Eggs are the best source of choline, and this mineral is required for a variety of processes in the human body, especially in the development of the brain. A survey conducted in the US showed that close to ninety percent of the people consumed very little choline. If you eat less choline, you will harm your fetus. A low intake can lead to decreased function in the brain of the fetus and also increase the risk of developing neural tube defects. One egg contains at least 113 milligrams of choline, and this covers at least twenty-five percent of the required intake.

Dark, Leafy Greens and Broccoli

Dark, leafy greens, like spinach and kale, and broccoli are rich in nutrients that every pregnant woman should consume. These nutrients include vitamin K, vitamin C, vitamin A, potassium, folate, iron and fiber. Leafy greens and broccoli have antioxidants and plant compounds that aid in digestion and improve the immune system. Since these vegetables are rich in fiber, they will help to prevent constipation. As mentioned earlier, this is a problem that most pregnant women face. You can also reduce the risk of low birth weight by increasing your intake of leafy vegetables.

· · ·

Lean Meat

Pork, chicken and beef are the best sources of lean protein. Pork and beef are rich in choline, vitamin B and iron, which are the nutrients that are required in abundance during pregnancy. Red blood cells require iron to increase the hemoglobin content. Hemoglobin is used to pass oxygen to every cell in your body. Since the blood volume increases during pregnancy, it is important for women to increase their intake of iron especially during the third trimester. Iron deficiency during the first trimester can increase the risk of low birth weight and premature delivery. Many women do not like meat during their pregnancy, and this makes it hard for them to consume the required amount of iron through their diet alone. For those who can eat meat, you should consume at least one serving of red meat on alternate days to increase the amount of iron that you acquire through your diet. The consumption of foods rich in vitamin C will help to improve your body's ability to absorb iron.

Fish Liver Oil

Fish liver oil is often extracted from the codfish. The oil is taken from the oily liver. This oil is rich in long chain omega-3 fatty acids like DHA and EPA. These are essential for the development of the eye and brain. Fish liver oil is rich in Vitamin D, and most people do not get enough of this vitamin. If you do not consume seafood, you will need to consume a vitamin D or Omega-3 supplement. Low vitamin D increases the risk of preeclampsia which is a complication today is potentially dangerous. This complication is characterized by the swelling of feet and hands, protein in the urine and high blood pressure. When you consume cod liver oil during the first few weeks of pregnancy, you can ensure that your baby has a high birth weight. One serving of this oil can help you meet your daily intake requirement of vitamin A, Vitamin D and omega-3 fatty acids. You should, however, ensure that you do not consume too much since that will lead to vitamin A toxicity in your body.

Berries

Berries are rich in Vitamin C, antioxidants and fiber, and are packed with healthy carbs and water. Vitamin C improves your body's ability to absorb iron, and this vitamin is also essential to improve the functioning of the immune system and maintain skin health. Berries do not cause any spikes in the blood sugar levels because they have a very low glycemic index. Since these fruits contain both fiber and water, they are a great snack, and they are nutritious and have a low number of calories.

Whole Grains

It is important for women to consume whole grains during their pregnancy since this helps them increase their intake of calories. Whole grains are rich in plant compounds, fiber and vitamins when compared to refined grains. Quinoa and oats contain a good amount of protein, and this nutrient is essential to consume during pregnancy since it helps to maintain and repair the tissues in the body. Whole grains are also rich in magnesium, Vitamin B and fiber.

Avocados

Avocados are probably the only fruit that is rich in mono-saturated fatty acids. This fruit is also rich in Vitamin K, Vitamin B, folate, Vitamin E, Vitamin C, copper, potassium and fiber. Since avocados are rich in potassium, healthy fats and folate, doctors and nutritionists advise women to consume avocados. The healthy fats help to build the brain, tissues and the skin of your fetus, and the folate reduces the risk of developing neural tube defects. One of the side effects of pregnancy is leg cramps, and potassium helps to relieve these cramps.

Dried Fruit

Dried fruit are rich in various vitamins, minerals and fiber, and high in calories. There is no difference between fresh fruit and dry fruit except for the fact that the latter has no water and is smaller in size. Therefore, you will consume the required intake of numerous vitamins and minerals including iron, potassium and folate when you consume one serving of dried fruit. Prunes are rich in Vitamin K, sorbitol, fiber and potassium, and they are natural laxatives. If you have constipation, you should consume at least one serving of this fruit every day. Dates are rich in potassium, plant compounds, fiber and iron, and it is important for women to consume dates regularly during the first and third trimesters since this will help to reduce the need for induced labor and also help to facilitate in the dilation of the cervix. Dried fruit also contains large quantities of natural sugar, and it is for this reason that you avoid the consumption of the candied dried fruit. Dried fruit does help to increase your intake of nutrients and calories, but doctors recommend that women consume only one serving of dried fruit per day during their pregnancy.

Water

The volume of blood will increase by 50 ounces during pregnancy, and it is important that you stay hydrated during your pregnancy. If you do not watch your intake of water, you will soon be dehydrated because your baby will get everything that he or she needs from you. Some symptoms of mild dehydration are anxiety, headaches, bad mood, reduced memory and tiredness. When you increase your intake of water, you can reduce the risk of urinary tract infections and also help to relieve constipation. These are common issues that women have during pregnancy. Women are advised to drink at least two liters of water every day during their pregnancy, but the amount varies for each individual. You should also bear in mind that you do get water from food and beverages like coffee, tea, vegetables and fruit. It is important that you drink water whenever you are thirsty, and drink the required amount of water to quench your thirst.

Chapter Four

UNHEALTHY FOODS EQUALS UNHEALTHY BABY

*I*t is a known fact that the most sensitive period or time in a woman's life is pregnancy, and it is important that women consume a healthy diet during that time. It is also important for women who are trying to get pregnant to consume a healthy diet. This chapter lists different foods that women should avoid during their pregnancy.

High-Mercury Fish

Mercury is one of the most toxic elements, and this element is often found in polluted water. There is no amount of Mercury that is considered safe. Large quantities of mercury are toxic to the kidneys, nervous system and immune system. Mercury can also lead to some developmental issues in children. Most marine fish have large amounts of mercury in their body, and it is for this reason that women are advised to consume only one or two servings of high-mercury fish per month during their pregnancy. Some fish that have high-mercury are:

- Tuna, especially albacore tuna
- Swordfish
- King mackerel
- Shark

It is, however, important for you to understand that every marine fish does not have too much mercury. It is only some types that have large quantities of mercury in their body. It is essential that you consume low-mercury fish during your pregnancy, and it is healthy to consume one serving of this fish at least twice a week.

Raw or Undercooked Fish

Raw fish can lead to several infections that can be parasitic, bacterial or viral like Salmonella, Vibrio, Listeria and norovirus. A few of these infections only affect the mother and often leave her weak and dehydrated. Some infections can pass on to the fetus and lead to serious, and sometimes fatal, consequences. Most women are vulnerable to the Listeria bacteria during their pregnancy. Studies show that pregnant women are twenty percent more likely to develop an infection caused by Listeria when compared to the general population. Listeria can be found in soil, polluted water and on contaminated fruit and vegetables. Raw fish is often infected by Listeria during smoking and drying. Mothers may not show any symptoms if they are affected by Listeria, but these bacteria will pass to the fetus through the placenta. This can lead to miscarriage, stillbirth, premature delivery and other health issues. It is for this reason that women are advised to avoid raw fish during their pregnancy. This means that you cannot consume sushi ever.

. . .

Raw, Processed and Undercooked Meat

You will increase the risk of developing infections from several parasites and bacteria, like Listeria, Salmonella, E.coli and Toxoplasma, if you eat raw or undercooked meat. The bacteria and parasites can threaten the health of your baby. If you are infected by any of these parasites, the risk of developing severe neurological illnesses or stillbirth increases. The risk of developing intellectual disabilities, epilepsy and blindness also increases. Most of the bacteria in meat is present on the surface and can easily be washed off. There are times when these bacteria are present inside the fibers of the muscles. You can consume the sirloins, ribeye and tenderloins of lamb, veal and beef even if they are not cooked fully. It is important to remember that this holds good only for the meat that is uncut or whole. Cut meat including burgers, meat patties, pork, minced meat and poultry should always be consumed when they are cooked fully. Deli meat, lunchmeat and hot dogs also must be consumed when fully cooked, because bacteria or parasites can contaminate them during storage or processing. It is for this reason that women should always consume processed meat products only when they are steaming hot.

Raw Eggs

Most raw eggs are contaminated with salmonella. Only the mother shows any symptoms of being affected by salmonella, and these symptoms include vomiting, nausea, fever, diarrhea and stomach cramps. However, these infections could lead to premature birth, stillbirth and terrible cramps in the uterus. Let us look at some foods that contain raw eggs:

- Homemade ice cream

- Homemade mayonnaise
- Poached eggs
- Lightly scrambled eggs
- Hollandaise sauce
- Salad dressings
- Cake icings

Commercial products often contain pasteurized raw eggs, and it is for this reason that you can consume these products during your pregnancy. Having said that, it is important that you always read the label to ensure that the eggs are pasteurized. It is important that you cook eggs or eat only pasteurized eggs.

Organ Meat

Organ meat is rich in vitamin B12, copper, iron and Vitamin A. These vitamins and minerals are essential for the health of the baby and the mother. That said, you should avoid the consumption of too much organ meat since that will increase the quantity of Vitamin A leading to toxicity in the body. Increased consumption of organ meat will increase the levels of copper in the body. This will result in liver toxicity and birth defects. It is for this reason that it is important that pregnant women do not consume more than one serving of organ meat per week.

Caffeine

One of the commonly used psychoactive substances is caffeine, and this substance is found in tea, coffees, cocoa and soft drinks. Doctors recommend that pregnant women limit their caffeine intake to only two cups of coffee a day. The body absorbs caffeine very quickly, and this compound quickly moves into the placenta. The levels of caffeine can build up inside the fetus and the placenta since neither has the enzyme that can break caffeine down. A high intake of caffeine can increase the risk of low birth weight and can also restrict the growth of the fetus. Low birth weight is directly linked to chronic diabetes, like heart disease and Type II diabetes, and infant death.

Raw Sprouts

Raw sprouts like clover, alfalfa, mung bean sprouts and radish are often contaminated with salmonella. These bacteria thrive in humid environments, and they are impossible to remove from the plants. It is for this reason that women are advised against the consumption of raw sprouts. Having said that, sprouts once cooked are safe to consume.

Unwashed Produce

Most vegetables and fruit are contaminated with several parasites and bacteria, including listeria, toxoplasma, Salmonella and E.coli. These bacteria and parasites can be acquired during handling or from the soil. It is important to remember that vegetables and fruit can get contaminated at any time during harvest, storage, production, retail and trans portation. Bacteria and parasites can harm both the baby and the mother. Toxoplasma is one of the most dangerous parasites that linger on vegetables and fruit. Most people who have invested toxoplasma do not show any symptoms, but there are a few people who do have a cold or the flu for more than a month. There are times when the fetus is infected with toxoplasma, but the symptoms, like intellectual disabilities and blindness, only appear later in life. Some babies may be born with serious brain or eye damage. So, when you are pregnant you should always rinse, peel and cook vegetables and fruit to reduce the risk of developing infections.

Unpasteurized Fruit Juice, Cheese and Milk

Unpasteurized and raw milk and cheese will contain some harmful bacteria including E.coli, Salmonella, Campylobacter and Listeria. The same can be said about unpasteurized juice since these juices can be contaminated easily. Any of these bacterial infections can lead to life-threatening consequences for your baby. Some of these bacterial are present in these foods, and they multiply due to contamination during storage or collection. One of the best ways to effectively kill these bacteria is through pasteurization. This process does not reduce the nutritional content of the products. It is for this reason that women are advised to drink pasteurized fruit juice, milk and cheese.

Alcohol

Doctors recommend that women should avoid alcohol during their pregnancy since alcohol increases the risk of still-birth and miscarriage. A small amount of alcohol can severely affect the development of your baby's brain, and can lead to fetal alcohol syndrome. As a result of this syndrome, your baby can develop intellectual disabilities, facial deformities and heart defects. There are no studies that can prove that small amounts of alcohol during pregnancy do not harm the mother or baby.

Processed Junk Food

During your pregnancy, you will notice that you and your baby are growing at a rapid rate. It is for this reason that you need to increase your intake of healthy nutrients including iron, protein and folate. It is true that you will be eating for two, but you do not need to double your caloric intake. As mentioned earlier, you will only need to increase your caloric intake by 450 calories. During your pregnancy, you will need to consume food that is rich in nutrients to ensure that you fulfill the needs of your body and your baby's. Processed junk food does not have any nutrients and is rich in added fats, sugar and calories. Studies show that added sugar can increase the risk of developing numerous diseases like heart disease and Type II Diabetes. It is necessary that you gain weight during pregnancy, but this excess weight gain can lead to different diseases, like gestational diabetes, and complications in birth. It can also increase the risk of giving birth to an overweight child, which will lead to some long-term health issues.

Chapter Five

SOME IMPORTANT TIPS

*I*t is important to ensure that you consume the right food during pregnancy to ensure the health of your baby. As mentioned earlier, when you consume the right food, you can reduce the risk of any illnesses or diseases that your child may develop after birth.

Eating for Two During Pregnancy

You will need to make sure that you change your eating habits during your pregnancy regardless of whether you were preparing to become pregnant or were surprised by the pregnancy. Numerous women start their pregnancy with a deficiency in numerous nutrients that are important for a healthy pregnancy. It is important that you meet the daily requirement of nutrients during your pregnancy since you will be eating for you and your baby. Research suggests that it is important for you to change your eating habits during your pregnancy since the food you eat then will determine the well-being of your child while he or she is in the womb, at birth and beyond birth. Your lifestyle will either increase or decrease the risk of your child developing numerous conditions like heart diseases, obesity and diabetes.

Always Focus on Folic Acid

You will have read repeatedly how important it is for you to consume folic acid during your pregnancy. Folic acid is one of the best ways to improve your child's health. As mentioned earlier, it is important for you to consume folic acid during the first trimester to reduce the risk of developing neural tube defects. It is important that you increase your intake of folic acid by consuming supplements. You should also consume fortified bread, cereal, pasta and rice.

Understand That Multivitamins Have Different Effects During Pregnancy

A multivitamin does not only provide the required nutrients for the mother and the baby, but has many other benefits. Studies show that prenatal vitamins and multivitamin tablets help to reduce the risk of preeclampsia, which increases the quantity of protein in the urine and increases blood pressure, by at least 40 percent. Preeclampsia can lead to premature birth or stillbirth. You may find it difficult to swallow your multivitamin tablets during pregnancy since these pills contain large quantities of iron that can cause constipation. These pills are also big which makes it difficult to swallow them. If you find that you have trouble with prenatal vitamins you should let your doctor know since you are having some unwanted side effects. Ensure that you let your doctor know about all the supplements that you are taking.

. . .

Always Make the Calories Count

It will be slightly difficult to monitor your weight gain during the first trimester. There are a few women who lose weight during this time since they have a lot of nausea and queasiness. This will prevent them from eating or drinking. If you are constantly nauseous or vomit often, you should consult your doctor because you will become dehydrated. Morning sickness often dissipates after the first few weeks of pregnancy, but you may feel nauseous throughout your pregnancy. When your baby begins to grow, you will need to increase your intake of calories by consuming food that is rich in nutrients. It is true that you will be eating for two people, but this does not mean that you can overeat. As mentioned earlier in the book, you will need to consume only 300 additional calories during your pregnancy. This may sound like a lot of calories. It is certainly okay to splurge on some hot chocolate or eat comfort food when you have cravings. You can make the additional calories that you consume in the following manner:

- 16 ounces of full fat or 1% low fat milk
- 2 ounces of chicken
- 1 teaspoon of mayonnaise
- 2 – 4 slices of whole-wheat bread
- 4 ounces non-fat or full-fast yogurt with fruit
- 1 ounce whole grain cereal

Weighty Matters During Pregnancy

It is important for you to gain the recommended number of pounds during your pregnancy to reduce any complications during delivery or pregnancy. Your weight will determine the health of your baby. Women who have a normal weight before they are pregnant will gain at least 35 pounds during pregnancy, but the weight will vary if they are giving birth to twins. It is important for women who are underweight or overweight to either gain more weight or lose weight before they become pregnant. If you were overweight before you became pregnant, you must ensure that you do not diet during your pregnancy. You should work closely with your dietician to ensure that you maintain your weight during your pregnancy.

Rethink Your Fluids During Pregnancy

You should ensure that you drink at least ten glasses of fluid every day during your pregnancy. You can drink plain water if you do not want to drink juice or milk. You should ensure that you do not consume any alcohol during your pregnancy since it can lead to some physical and mental defects in the baby. In the third and fourth chapter of the book, you will gather information about the different types of fluids that you can and cannot drink during your pregnancy.

CONCLUSION

Thank you for purchasing the book.

Pregnancy is one of the most cherished times in a woman's life. Having said that, it is also one of the most sensitive periods in a woman's life because she will need to take care of herself and her child. You will, therefore, need to ensure that you consume the right food to improve your health and also aid in the growth and development of the fetus.

Over the course of the book, you will have gathered information about the different foods that you should consume during pregnancy and also the list of foods you should avoid. If you follow the instructions given in the book word for word, you can ensure that you and your baby are healthy.

SOURCES

https://www.webmd.com/baby/features/top-tips-
pregnancy-nutrition#4

https://www.ncbi.nlm.nih.gov/pmc/articles/PMC6413112/

https://www.johnmuirhealth.com/health-education/health-
wellness/pregnancy-breastfeeding/nutritional-needs-during-
pregnancy.html

https://www.ncbi.nlm.nih.gov/pmc/articles/PMC5084016/

https://www.healthline.com/nutrition/11-foods-to-avoid-
during-pregnancy

https://www.healthline.com/nutrition/13-foods-to-eat-when-
pregnant

https://www.mayoclinic.org/healthy-lifestyle/pregnancy-week-
by-week/in-depth/pregnancy-nutrition/art-20045082

https://www.livescience.com/45090-pregnancy-diet.html

FOOD FOR PREGNANCY VOLUME 2

*The Moms Guide to Understanding the Best Supplements
and Nutrients for a Healthy Growing Baby*

INTRODUCTION

Pregnancy is a time of anticipation and excitement, but a few women experience some complications like anemia, high blood pressure or bleeding during their pregnancy. There are several other complications that they may experience during pregnancy.

In the first volume, you learnt about the different nutrients that you must consume during pregnancy, and when you are deficient in any of those nutrients, there are higher chances of there being complications during delivery. Over the course of this book, you will gather information on the different complications that women experience during pregnancy due to deficiencies or otherwise. You will also gather information on what women can do to prevent these complications.

Since most complications arise due to a deficiency in an important nutrient, you will need to take supplements. This book also sheds some light on the different supplements you can take to prevent the deficiency. You will also gather information about the different exercises you can perform to make it easier for you during pregnancy and during birth. It is important that you are cautious when you perform these exercises so you can avoid any complications in the future. There are some tests that you are required to take during your pregnancy to ensure the health of your baby and yourself. These tests have been listed in this book.

Thank you for purchasing the book. I hope you gather all the information you are looking for.

Chapter One

SUPPLEMENTS TO TAKE DURING PREGNANCY

*P*regnancy is a very happy experience and one of the most exciting times in a woman's life. However, it can be overwhelming and confusing for some women. Numerous advertisements, magazines and articles on the Internet advise a woman on how she should stay healthy during her pregnancy. Women are aware that they should never smoke, drink alcohol or consume high-mercury seafood during their pregnancy. But few are aware that some vitamins, herbal supplements and minerals must be avoided as well. It becomes very complicated to identify those supplements which are safe and which are not safe to take during pregnancy since this information varies between the sources. This chapter will shed some light on the different supplements that you can take and those you should avoid during your pregnancy.

Why Take Supplements During Pregnancy?

It is important that you consume the right nutrients at every stage of your life, but it is especially important to consume these nutrients during your pregnancy since a pregnant woman will need to nourish their body and also aid in the development of the fetus.

• *Pregnancy Increases the Need for Nutrients*

A woman will need to increase her intake of macronutrients during pregnancy, and these macronutrients include fats, carbohydrates and proteins. This has been covered in detail in the first volume of the book. The requirement of the micronutrients will increase by a large quantity during pregnancy. Vitamins and minerals help to support the fetal and maternal growth at every stage in the pregnancy. These nutrients are important to support some critical functions like cell signaling and cell growth. Some women find it easy to meet these growing needs through their diets, while others cannot. These women will need to take supplements for various reasons including:

1. To prevent nutrient deficiencies, some women may have some deficiencies in the essential vitamins and minerals, and it is important to correct these deficiencies. A shortage in the nutrients can lead to numerous complications during pregnancy and birth defects.
2. To prevent severe vomiting and nausea. This condition is called hyperemesis gravidarum, and can lead to nutrient deficiencies and weight loss.
3. To prevent micronutrient deficiencies caused due to following specific diets. Some women consume a vegan or vegetarian diet because they have some food allergies and intolerances. They need to take supplements to prevent these deficiencies.

4. To cater for the increased need of folate and Vitamin C. Some women find it difficult to quit smoking even during pregnancy, and this will increase their need for folate and vitamin C.

5. To ensure the optimal nutrition for both the mother and her babies if the mother is carrying more than one baby. When a woman is carrying multiple babies, she will need to increase her nutrient intake so she can provide adequate nutrition to the babies.

6. If a woman consumes a poor diet, or finds it difficult to consume the right foods she will need to take some supplements to avoid any deficiencies in vitamins or minerals.

Some experts from the American Congress of Obstetrics and Gynecology advise all pregnant women to take folic acid supplements and prenatal vitamins during their pregnancy. These supplements will help to prevent any birth defects or deficiencies. It is for this reason that mothers often take supplements.

• *Herbal Supplements During Pregnancy*

During pregnancy, women do not necessarily have to take vitamin or mineral supplements. They can also take herbal supplements. A study found that close to 15.4% women in the US used herbal supplements during their pregnancy. Close to 25% of these women did not consult their doctors when they were taking these supplements. Some herbal supplements can be taken during pregnancy, but there are others that are bad for women during their pregnancy. Some herbs do help with lowering the risk of complications during pregnancy like an upset stomach or nausea. However, some herbal supplements are harmful for both the mother and the fetus. There is very little research that talks about the benefits of using herbal supplements.

Supplements Considered Safe during Pregnancy

Just like any medication that you take, any herbal or micronutrient supplements you take during your pregnancy should be taken under your doctor's supervision. This is to ensure that you take the supplements in the safe amounts. You should always purchase these supplements from the right brands, so that the supplements are of high quality and are safe to take.

- *Prenatal Vitamins*

Every woman is advised to take prenatal vitamins during her pregnancy, and these vitamins have been formulated to meet the increased demand of these nutrients during pregnancy. These vitamins should be taken before you conceive the baby and during your pregnancy. Some studies show that prenatal vitamins help to reduce the risk of premature birth and preeclampsia. The latter is a dangerous complication that is caused due to high blood pressure and protein in the blood. Prenatal vitamins are not sued to replace a healthy diet, but they will help to prevent any deficiencies since they provide the pregnant woman with the required nutrients. Some prenatal vitamins contain minerals and vitamins that a woman would need to consume during her pregnancy. You will not need to take any other supplements unless advised by your doctor. Some prenatal vitamins that are prescribed by your doctor or midwife will be available over the counter.

- *Folate*

Folate is a Vitamin B, which plays an important role in the synthesis of DNA, production of red blood cells and the growth and development of the fetus. Folic acid is found in many supplements and this is the synthetic form of the folate mineral. This acid will be converted in L-methylfolate, which is the active form of folate. Nutritionists and doctors recommend that women increase their intake of folate up to 600 ug per day. This will help to reduce the risk of developing congenital abnormalities and neural tube defects. Adequate quantities of folate are obtained through the diet, but many women do not eat the required quantity of folate-rich foods. This makes it important for them to take supplements.

- *Iron*

Women will require more iron during their pregnancy since the volume of blood will increase by fifty percent during pregnancy. Iron is a mineral that is essential for the healthy development and growth of the placenta and fetus. This mineral is also important to transfer oxygen throughout the body. Most women are deficient in iron during their pregnancy, and anemia during pregnancy is associated with infant anemia, premature birth and maternal depression. It is recommended that women consume at least 27 mg of iron every day, and women can obtain this amount of iron through prenatal vitamins. Having said that, women with anemia or iron deficiency would need to consume higher doses. If you are not deficient in iron, you should not consume more than the required amount of iron to avoid any side effects including abnormally high hemoglobin levels, constipation and vomiting.

- *Vitamin D*

Vitamin D is a fat-soluble vitamin, which is used by the body to maintain bone health, improve the function of the immune system and aid in cell division. Any deficiency in this vitamin can lead to preeclampsia, gestational diabetes, preterm birth and cesarean section during birth. It is recommended that women take at least 600 IU of Vitamin D per day. Having said that, some experts suggest women require more Vitamin D during their pregnancy. You should always speak to your doctor about your intake of Vitamin D during your pregnancy.

- *Magnesium*

Magnesium is an important mineral that women should consume during their pregnancy. This mineral is an enzyme used in most chemical reactions that take place in your body, and also plays a critical role in nerve, immune and muscle function. If you are deficient in this mineral, it can increase the risk of premature labor and hypertension. Some studies suggest taking magnesium supplements will help to reduce the risk of any complications like premature birth and fetal growth restriction.

- *Ginger*

Ginger is a root that is often used as an herbal supplement and a spice. Ginger is often used as a supplement to reduce nausea, which is caused due to chemotherapy, motion sickness or pregnancy. Ginger is both effective and safe to treat vomiting and nausea that are caused due to pregnancy. Women will be nauseous and vomit during the first trimester, and sometimes they may also experience severe nausea throughout the pregnancy. Ginger will help to reduce this complication, but there is still some research that needs to be conducted to identify the safe dosage of this root.

- *Fish Oil*

If you remember from the first volume, we talked about how fish oil contains the two essential fatty acids EPA and DHA. These oils are important for the development of the brain of the fetus. You can take EPA and DHA supplements to boost the development of the fetus's brain and reduce the risk of maternal depression. There is yet some research that needs to be performed to confirm this. Some studies show EPA and DHA help to improve cognitive function in babies. For instance, one study that was conducted used 2399 women, but there was no difference that could be found in the cognitive development between the infants of mothers who used fish oil supplements and the infants of mothers who did not take any fish oil supplements. This study also concluded that there was no strong effect of this supplement on maternal depression. The study, however, did find that fish oil supplements did help to reduce the risk of premature birth and also helped in the development of the fetus's eyes. It is important for the mother to maintain the required DHA levels in her body to ensure that the fetus develops well. Pregnant women are advised to consume at least two or three servings of low-mercury fish like pollock, sardines and salmon every week.

- *Probiotics*

Since it is important for women to maintain their gut health during their pregnancy, they turn towards probiotics. Probiotics are living microorganisms that benefit the health of the digestive system. Many studies show that it is safe for women to take probiotics during their pregnancy, and there are no side effects that have been identified yet, except for the risk of some infection that can be caused due to probiotics. Numerous studies show supplementing your diet with probiotics will reduce the risk of developing postpartum depression, dermatitis, gestational diabetes and infant eczema. Research is still ongoing on the use of probiotics during pregnancy, and the effects of probiotics on fetal and maternal health are to be discovered.

Supplements to Avoid During Pregnancy

It is important that you supplement your body with some micronutrients or herbs, but there are some that you should avoid.

- *Vitamin A*

Vitamin A is important for the development of the fetus's immune system and vision, but too much Vitamin A can lead to toxicity in the body. The body stores excess Vitamin A in the liver, which accumulates in the body and leads to liver damage. It can also cause some birth defects. For instance, excess amounts of Vitamin A in the body is known to cause some congenital birth defects in babies. Pregnant women will get enough Vitamin A from their diet and through prenatal vitamins, and it is for this reason that they are advised to not take any supplements.

- *Vitamin E*

Vitamin E is a fat-soluble vitamin, which plays numerous

roles in the body, and it is involved in improving the function of the immune system and gene expression. This vitamin is important for health, but women are advised to never take vitamin E supplements during their pregnancy. Vitamin E supplements do not improve the health for both the mother and the baby, and can lead to abdominal pain or rupture the amniotic sack.

• *Black Cohosh*

Block cohosh is a plant that is used for numerous reasons including controlling menstrual cramps or hot flashes. This herb is a member of the buttercup family, and it is unsafe to take this herb during pregnancy since it can lead to premature birth or miscarriage because it causes uterine contractions. This herb is also known to cause some liver damage.

• *Goldenseal*

Goldenseal is a plant that is used to treat diarrhea and respiratory infections. It is a dietary supplement, but there is very little evidence that can confirm the safety and the effects of the herb on the body. This herb contains a substance termed berberine, which is known to cause more harm to infants, and can lead to the development of a condition called kernicterus. This condition can lead to brain damage or death. It is for this reason that women are advised to avoid this herb during pregnancy.

• *Dong quai*

Dong quai is a popular medicinal root used in Chinese medicine for over a thousand years. It is used to treat numerous issues right from high blood pressure to menstrual cramps, but there is very little evidence which suggests that this herb is safe to use during pregnancy or even otherwise. It is important that you avoid using this herb during your pregnancy since it can increase the risk of miscarriage since it stimulates uterine contractions.

- ***Yohimbe***

Yohimbe is a supplement that is obtained from the bark of a tree native to Africa. This supplement is an herbal remedy used to treat numerous conditions like obesity and erectile dysfunction. It is important that you never use this herb during your pregnancy because it is associated with numerous side effects like heart attacks, seizures and blood pressure.

- ***Herbal Supplements Considered Unsafe During Pregnancy***

Some supplements that you should avoid are:

1. Red clover
2. Saw palmetto
3. Pennyroyal
4. Tansy
5. Wormwood
6. Yarrow
7. Mugwort
8. Blue Cohosh
9. Angelica
10. Ephedra

Chapter Two

ANEMIA IN PREGNANCY

A few women become anemic during their pregnancy. This means that the number of red blood cells decreases in their body. Anemia will make you very tired during your pregnancy, but there are some ways in which you can manage it. If you are anemic during your pregnancy, you will be very tired than usual.

What Are Red Blood Cells?

The cells in your body are called red blood cells, and their role is to transport oxygen through your body. The oxygen is often carried from the heart to your brain, skin, muscles, kidney and every other part of your body. These cells are produced in the marrow in your bones. The red blood cells can carry the oxygen across the body because of the protein hemoglobin. If you want to ensure that you have enough hemoglobin in your body, you will need to consume Vitamin B12, folate and iron. These nutrients help the body produce the hemoglobin that it needs.

. . .

What Is Anemia?

You are anemic if your body does not have the required number of red blood cells in it to carry oxygen to your baby and all around your body. It is common to be mildly anemic during pregnancy, and if you are slightly anemic during pregnancy, you will be a little tired. If you have severe anemia, you will constantly be out of breath and will be terribly weak, irritable, and dizzy and may also find it very hard to concentrate on any task that you are performing. You will also find that your heart races every time.

Why Do Women Become Anemic During Pregnancy?

When a woman is pregnant, her body will change. These changes are necessary for promoting the growth of the baby. When you are pregnant, your body will need to make a lot more blood. A woman who is not pregnant will have close to five liters of blood in her body, but when she is pregnant, she will have at least eight liters of blood in her body. The body needs a lot of folate, iron and Vitamin B12 to increase the number of cells in the body, and also produce the extra hemoglobin. Anemia is mainly caused due to iron deficiency during pregnancy. When you are pregnant, you must remember to consume at least three times the amount of iron that you would consume when you are menstruating. It is unfortunately hard for the body to absorb iron, and this makes it harder to produce hemoglobin. It is for this reason that women are at a higher risk of being anemic during pregnancy.

Tests for Anemia

When you find out you are pregnant and go to visit the doctor or midwife, you will be asked to take a blood test which will help them understand your hemoglobin level. If there are any abnormalities in this test, you may need to take more tests to check the levels of folate, iron and Vitamin B12 in your body. You may also need to take a few tests that will shed some light on inherited disorders.

Risks Associated With Anemia during Pregnancy

Most women are tired during their pregnancy, but anemia worsens this condition. It will make you feel breathless and tired. The probability of you requiring a blood transfusion once you give birth to your baby will increase. Anemia can increase the risk of low birth weight and premature birth, and there is also a possibility that your child may be anemic.

How Can I Avoid Anemia During Pregnancy?

You can avoid anemia during pregnancy in the following ways:

- Always start your pregnancy in good health
- Make sure that you eat the right foods during pregnancy
- Take supplements if required

#1 *Starting Pregnancy In Great Health*

If you are trying to become pregnant, you should first meet with your doctor and get a full body check-up done. You will need to ask your doctor to shed some light on some conditions like anemia, and also ask your doctor about the supplements you may need to take for folate. Doctors often advise women to take a folate supplement for one month before they become pregnant, and continue to take that supplement until the end of the first trimester. This helps to reduce the risk of spina bifida and other neural tube defects. Women are advised to take at least 0.5 milligrams of folic acid every day during their pregnancy, but this amount varies if the woman is pregnant. Ensure that you always discuss your conditions with your doctor to avoid worsening the situation.

#2 *Eating Well During Pregnancy*

As mentioned in the first volume of the book, it is important that you eat the right food. You can lower the risk of being anemic by consuming foods that are rich in iron, like iron fortified cereals and breads, spinach, egg, dried fruit and meat. Vitamin B_{12} is found in dairy products, eggs, shellfish, meat and fish. Leafy green vegetables, muesli, beans, beef, broccoli, asparagus and Brussels sprouts are rich in folic acid, and it is advised that you consume these foods to lower the risk of anemia. If you are a vegetarian, you should replace the meat and fish with beans, lentils, soymilk, eggs and tofu. You should also meet with a dietician to learn more about how you can improve your nutrition, and also gather information about the different supplements you may need to take. It is best to avoid tea and coffee immediately after a meal, and also consume citrus fruit to improve your body's ability to absorb the iron that is found in the food you consume. This will help to prevent anemia.

#3 *Supplements*

Women are advised to take some supplements for folic acid during their pregnancy, and they are also advised to consume food that is rich in folate. Many women are required to take iron supplements especially when they are at a higher risk of becoming deficient or are deficient. Vegans and vegetarians are often asked to take supplements for the B12 vita-min, and if you have been asked to take those supplements you should speak to your doctor to learn about the side effects of supplements, and what you should do to avoid them.

Chapter Three

BLEEDING DURING PREGNANCY

It is common for women to bleed during their pregnancy, but any signs of vaginal bleeding are dangerous. If you notice that you are bleeding from the vagina, you should consult your doctor or midwife immediately. It is important to identify the cause of bleeding immediately, although it is not caused because of any serious issues. If you notice that you are bleeding from your vagina, you should contact your doctor immediately. There is a possibility that you may have some light bleeding during the first few weeks into your pregnancy, and this is called spotting. You bleed at this time since the fetus would have planted itself in the walls of the uterus. This bleeding is also termed as implantation bleeding, and will happen around the time of the first period after you have conceived.

Causes Of Bleeding

Vaginal bleeding during the first two months of pregnancy can be a sign of ectopic pregnancy or miscarriage. Ectopic pregnancy is the condition where the fetus implants itself in the fallopian tube. That said, many women who have had vaginal bleeding during this stage do have successful pregnancies and give birth to healthy babies. Vaginal bleeding can be caused due to other causes during the next few months of pregnancy. Some of the causes have been listed in this section.

#1 *Changes In The Cervix*

If you have sex during pregnancy, the cells in the cervix will change. They will become more sensitive and can cause bleeding. This condition is called cervical ectropion, which is a harmless condition. Quite often you may develop vaginal infections, which can lead to bleeding.

#2 *'Show'*

Show is the small quantity of blood that is mixed with the mucus. Most women have this sort of bleeding in the last trimester. During pregnancy, there is a plug of mucus that covers or seals the cervix. The mucus will mix with the blood when the plug comes away. This means that the cells in the cervix are changing, and your body is getting ready to enter the first stages of labor. This type of bleeding will occur either during labor or a few days before you go into labor.

#3 *Placental Abruption*

Placental Abruption is a very serious condition where the placenta will start to come away from the wall of the womb. This condition does not necessarily lead to vaginal bleeding, but will cause a stomach pain. You may give birth to your baby earlier if this condition occurs a few days before the due date.

#4 *Placenta Praevia*

Placenta Praevia, also termed low-lying placenta is a condition where the placenta is very close to the cervix or covering it, since it is attached to the lower section of the womb. This will make it difficult for your baby to come out of your body. You can check the position of your placenta in the morphology scan. The baby will not be able to move past the placenta if it is covering or close to the cervix. In these conditions, the doctor will recommend that you have a caesarean.

#5 *Vasa Praevia*

Vasa Praevia is a condition that occurs when the blood vessels in the umbilical cord cover the service through the membranes. This condition occurs in about 1 in 3000 to 1 in 6000 births. The blood vessels in the umbilical cord are often protected within the membrane of the cord, but if the membrane ruptures and your water breaks at the same time, these vessels can tear. This will lead to vaginal bleeding, and there is a chance that your baby may lose a lot of blood and die. It is difficult to identify the symptoms of vasa Praevia that makes it hard to diagnose. That being said, an ultrasound could help to spot this condition before birth. If the baby's heart rate suddenly changes, either drops or becomes rapid, or there is some bleeding in the vagina, you should ask your doctor to check for vasa Praevia. This condition is linked with placenta Praevia.

How to Identify the Causes of Bleeding?

You will need to have an ultrasound scan, a vaginal or pelvic examination or a blood test to check the hormone levels to identify the reason behind vaginal bleeding. You will also be asked about some other symptoms like dizziness, pain, cramps and more. If your baby is not due for a long time and the symptoms are not severe, the doctor will monitor you and may keep you under observation for a few days. Depending on what is causing the bleeding, you may need to stay in the hospital only for one night or until you give birth. This is to keep you and your baby healthy, and deliver your baby safely regardless of what the situation may be.

Chapter Four

ITCHING DURING PREGNANCY

*Y*ou may have some mild itching during your pregnancy since your blood will supply more blood to the skin. The skin around your abdomen will also be stretched during your pregnancy as your baby grows, and this may also feel slightly itchy. You do not have to worry about mild itching, but if the itching becomes severe it could be a sign of obstetric cholestasis, which is a liver condition. Only one pregnant woman out of 100 will be affected by this condition.

Mild itching

You can wear loose clothes to prevent any itching since your clothes will not cause any friction by rubbing against your skin. This will reduce any irritation. You should try to wear only cotton or other natural fabrics to ensure that air will circulate across your body. You may also feel relief when you apply some moisturizer or lotion or take a cool bath. If you find that some strong perfumes irritate your skin, you should switch to mild perfumes. If you have severe itching,

which does not stop, you should consult your doctor immediately.

Obstetric Cholestasis (OC)

Obstetric cholestasis (OC) or intrahepatic cholestasis is a
liver disorder, which only affects some women during pregnancy, especially in the last trimester.

#1 Causes Of Obstetric Cholestasis

The causes of OC are still unclear. In some cases, the pregnancy hormone can also be involved. Since the pregnancy
hormones increase in the body during pregnancy, these
hormones will reduce the flow of bile. This means that the
number of salts in the bile will add up in the liver instead of
leaving it. These salts will enter the bloodstream, which will
make you feel itchy.

OC often runs in families, but it can occur during pregnancy even if you do not have any family that has been
affected by this disorder. If you did have OC in a previous
pregnancy, you may also develop it during your subsequent
pregnancies. If you have OC, the risk of premature birth and
stillbirth increases. Your baby may also have some issues with
breathing, and your doctor may induce labor even before your
due date to prevent these complications.

#2 Symptoms Of Obstetric Cholestasis

One of the classic symptoms of OC is an itch without any
rash. This usually happens on the soles of your feet and your
palms, but some times it can be more widespread. The
itching will become worse at night and is also unbearable and

continuous. Another symptom of OC is jaundice, pale bowel movements and dark urine. You will find that the itchiness has gone after you gave birth.

#3 *Treating Obstetric Cholestasis*

Obstetric cholestasis can be diagnosed based on family and medical history. You can also take some blood tests to check the functioning of the liver. If you are diagnosed with OG, you will need to have liver function tests regularly until you give birth. These tests will allow the doctor to closely monitor your condition. Calamine lotion and other creams prescribed by your doctor can be used during pregnancy. These creams can provide some relief. Your doctor may also ask you to take some medication that reduces itching and decreases the number of bile salts. OC will make it difficult for your body to absorb Vitamin K, which is an important nutrient to ensure that blood clots. Discuss your options and your health with your doctor or midwife if you are diagnosed with OC.

Chapter Five

HIGH BLOOD PRESSURE DURING PREGNANCY

*I*t is said that you have high blood pressure if the measure of your blood pressure is either equal to or greater than 130/80 mm Hg. This condition is serious and is a major concern for many women. If it is managed well, high blood pressure does not necessarily have to be dangerous during pregnancy.

Causes of High Blood Pressure during Pregnancy

There are numerous reasons why a woman may develop high blood pressure during her pregnancy, and these include:

- Being obese or overweight
- Not keeping yourself active
- Drinking alcohol
- Smoking
- First-time pregnancy
- History of hypertension in the family
- Age is over 35
- Multiple births

• Having autoimmune diseases like diabetes

Risk Factors

There are some risk factors that lead to high blood pressure during pregnancy.

#1 Pregnancy

Women who are pregnant for the first time will most likely have high blood pressure, but there is a chance that this condition will not arise during future pregnancies. If a woman is carrying multiple babies, it can lead to hypertension. The woman's body will need to twice or thrice as hard to ensure that it provides the required nourishment to the babies.

#2 Lifestyle

An unhealthy lifestyle can increase the risk of developing hypertension or high blood pressure during pregnancy. If you are obese or overweight, or not keeping yourself active, the risk of developing high blood pressure will increase.

#3 Age

Pregnant women who are above the age of thirty-five are at a higher risk of developing hypertension. Women who have hypertension before they become pregnant will be at a higher risk of developing some complications during pregnancy when compared to those women who have normal blood pressure before they become pregnant.

. . .

Different Blood Related Conditions

There are three different conditions that a woman can develop during pregnancy if she has hypertension.

#1 Chronic hypertension

Many times women have hypertension or high blood pressure before they become pregnant. This condition is also known as chronic hypertension and can be treated with medication. Doctors also say that women who develop hypertension during their pregnancy have chronic hypertension, and this is true for those women who develop hypertension during the first twenty weeks of their pregnancy.

#2 Gestational hypertension

You can develop gestational hypertension during your twentieth week of pregnancy, and this condition will resolve after delivery. If gestational hypertension is diagnosed before thirty weeks, it can increase the risk of developing preeclampsia.

#3 Superimposed Preeclampsia And Chronic Hypertension

If you had chronic hypertension before you became pregnant, you will develop preeclampsia during your pregnancy. This can lead to some additional complications during pregnancy including protein in your urine.

Checking Your Blood Pressure

The blood pressure is measured as a fraction where the

systolic blood pressure is the numerator and the diastolic blood pressure is the denominator. The systolic blood pressure will measure the pressure of blood in your arteries when your heart is squeezing or beating the blood from the heart to your body. The diastolic pressure will measure the pressure of blood in your arteries when your heart is at rest.

You do not have to go to the doctor to track your blood pressure, but can purchase a blood pressure monitor online or from the pharmacy. Most of these devices will be placed only on your upper arm or wrist. You can take the monitor to your doctor's office to help you check the accuracy of the monitor. You can also visit any store including a grocery store or pharmacy where you can take the blood pressure readings. You should take the readings of the blood pressure at the same time every day to ensure that you have accurate readings. Keep your legs uncrossed and always use the same arm. If you have high blood pressure repeatedly, you should inform your doctor immediately.

#1 Normal Blood Pressure

Your doctor will take a baseline measurement of your blood pressure at the start of your pregnancy to determine what your normal blood pressure during pregnancy should be. They will then measure the blood pressure during every visit.

#2 High Blood Pressure

If your blood pressure is greater than 130/99 mm Hg, or you are at a higher number than the pressure before you became pregnant, you will need to visit the doctor immediately. High blood pressure is defined as a high systolic with a diastolic that is 90 mm Hg or higher or the pressure is 140 mm Hg. The blood pressure may decrease for a woman early in pregnancy, since the pregnancy hormones will lead to the widening of the blood vessels, and as a result of this the flow of blood in the body will not be too high.

#3 *Low Blood Pressure*

There is no number that you can put to determine low blood pressure. The following are some symptoms of low blood pressure:

- Cold and clammy skin
- Headache
- Feeling Faint
- Dizziness
- Nausea

What Causes Changes in Blood Pressure?

When a woman progresses through her pregnancy, the blood pressure can return to the normal level or change depending on your body. Here are some reasons behind why this may happen.

1. The quantity of blood will increase in the body. Numerous studies conclude that a woman's blood volume will increase by forty-five percent during pregnancy, and this extra blood will need to be pumped throughout the body by the heart.
2. The left side of the heart, which does the pumping, will become larger and thicker. This will give the heart a chance to pump more blood.
3. The kidneys will increase the production of the

hormone vasopressin, which will lead to water
retention in the body.

High blood pressure during pregnancy will often reduce
when you give birth to the baby. In some situations, the blood
pressure will continue to be elevated and your doctor will
prescribe some medication to bring the level back to normal.

Chapter Six

PREECLAMPSIA

any women develop preeclampsia during their pregnancy after twenty weeks. They may also develop preeclampsia immediately after they deliver their baby. If you have preeclampsia, you will have fluid retention or edema, high blood pressure and some protein in the urine. If you do not treat this immediately, it can lead to some severe complications, and can be life threatening in some instances. Preeclampsia can lead to growth and development problems in the baby.

The exact cause of preeclampsia is still unknown, but it is thought that preeclampsia occurs whenever there is an issue with the placenta. Women may not realize that they have preeclampsia during their pregnancy, and it can only be diagnosed through routine appointments with the doctor or midwife.

Pre-eclampsia symptoms

#1 Early Symptoms

Women who develop preeclampsia will show the following symptoms:

- Protein in the urine or proteinuria
- Hypertension or high blood pressure

You will not notice these symptoms during your pregnancy, but your midwife or doctor should pick these up during your appointments. Most pregnant women suffer from high blood pressure, so this cannot suggest preeclampsia. If there is protein in your urine, it can be used to indicate the condition.

#2 *Progressive Symptoms*

When you develop preeclampsia, it will lead to retention of fluid. This will cause swelling in the ankles, feet, hands and face. Fluid retention or edema is a common symptom of pregnancy, but it will only happen in the lower parts of the body like the ankles and the feet. Edema will gradually develop, but if the swelling is very sudden it can be a sign of preeclampsia. Preeclampsia may cause the following as it progresses:

- Less urine
- Vision problems, such as seeing flashing lights or blurring
- Feeling generally unwell
- Nausea and vomiting
- Excessive weight gain
- Dizziness
- Severe headaches
- Shortness of breath
- Pain in the upper abdomen (just below the ribs)

When you notice any of these symptoms, you should meet your doctor immediately. Preeclampsia can lead to numerous complications if it is not treated properly. Some of these complications are:

- HELLP (a combination of blood-clotting and liver disorder)
- Stroke
- Eclampsia (convulsions)
- Problems in the kidneys and brain

These complications are, however, extremely rare.

How Does Preeclampsia Affect Your Unborn Baby?

Preeclampsia can lead to premature birth of your baby, and one of the main signs of preeclampsia is slow growth of the fetus. The fetus will not receive adequate blood supply through the placenta, and the fetus will also receive fewer nutrients and less oxygen, which are essential for the growth of the baby. This condition is termed as intra-uterine growth retardation or intra-uterine growth restriction.

Risk factors

Some factors have been identified which can increase the risk of developing preeclampsia. Some of them are:

- You developed preeclampsia during your previous pregnancy which means that there is a twenty percent probability that you will develop this condition in future pregnancies.

- You have high blood pressure, migraines, diabetes and kidney disease.

Some of the other risk factors are:

- There are higher chances of you developing preeclampsia during your first pregnancy when compared to your future pregnancies.
- Your last pregnancy was over ten years ago.
- Either your mother or sister had preeclampsia during their pregnancy.
- You are either aged over 40 or are a teenager.
- You were obese before your pregnancy.
- You are having twins or triplets.

Treating preeclampsia

You can treat preeclampsia by maintaining your blood pressure and treating the other symptoms through medication. One of the simplest ways to treat preeclampsia is to give birth to the baby.

Chapter Seven

SEVERE VOMITING DURING PREGNANCY

*V*omiting and nausea are very common during pregnancy, and this is especially true during the first trimester. Some women experience excessive vomiting and nausea, and this condition is called hyperemesis gravidarum. You will need to be treated by a doctor if you suffer from this condition. This condition is not very common, but it can be treated. It is worse than morning sickness, and if you are unable to keep any food or fluids down, you should tell your doctor or midwife immediately.

Symptoms of hyperemesis gravidarum

If you have excessive vomiting during your pregnancy, you will find that it is much worse than morning sickness or nausea. The symptoms of excessive vomiting will start five weeks into your pregnancy, and will resolve by the twentieth week. Some of the signs of hyperemesis gravidarum are:

- Ketosis, which is a serious condition that is caused

due to an increase in the number of ketones in the urine and blood. Ketones are acidic chemicals that are produced by your body when it breaks down fat to produce energy.

- Severe or prolonged vomiting and nausea
- Weight loss
- Dehydration
- Confusion, jaundice, fainting and headaches
- Hypotension or low blood pressure when you stand up

The vomiting or nausea is often so severe that it becomes impossible for you to keep any food or fluids in your stomach. This will lead to weight loss and dehydration. Hyperemesis gravidarum is often unpleasant and has some dramatic symptoms. The good news is that it will not harm your baby. That being said, if you lose too much weight during pregnancy there is a risk of low birth weight.

Treating hyperemesis gravidarum

Some cases of hyperemesis gravidarum can be controlled using antacids, through rest and through a change in diet. Some severe cases of hyperemesis gravidarum will require special treatment, and you will need to be admitted in the hospital so that your doctor can asses the condition and give you the required treatment. You may be given some intravenous fluids through a drip to stop the vomiting and also treat the ketosis. You should never take any medication without speaking to your doctor first.

Blood clots and hyperemesis gravidarum

Since hyperemesis gravidarum can lead to dehydration, you are at a higher risk of developing a blood clot or deep being thrombosis.

Chapter Eight

GESTATIONAL DIABETES DURING PREGNANCY

*I*f you have high levels of blood sugar during your pregnancy, you have gestational diabetes. Your blood sugar levels may have been normal before you became pregnant, but they may have increased during your pregnancy. Having said that, you could still give birth to a healthy baby even if you have gestational diabetes. You should visit your doctor and take some simple steps that will help you manage your blood sugar levels. When you baby is born, you will see that the gestational diabetes goes away. The risk of developing Type II diabetes after you give birth increases if you have gestational diabetes.

Symptoms of Gestational Diabetes

There are no symptoms of gestational diabetes in women, and many women only learn that they have gestational diabetes when they go through their routine tests.

What Causes Gestational Diabetes?

The placenta produces hormones during pregnancy, and these hormones can increase the quantity of glucose in your blood. The pancreas will produce enough insulin, which can handle this increase in glucose, but if your body cannot produce the required quantity of insulin, the blood sugar levels will increase. This will lead to the development of gestational diabetes.

Risk Factors for Gestational Diabetes

Gestational diabetes affects at least ten percent of pregnancy each year, and you may develop gestational diabetes if you:

- Are Asian, African-American, Native American or Hispanic
- Were overweight before you were pregnant
- Have a family history of diabetes
- Have very high blood sugar levels, but this does not necessarily lead to diabetes
- Have some medical complications including high blood pressure
- Have given birth to a baby who weighed greater than nine pounds
- Have given birth to a baby with birth defects or a stillborn baby
- Are older than 25
- Have had gestational diabetes in previous pregnancies

Gestational Diabetes Tests and Diagnosis

It is only after twelve weeks that the risk of gestational

diabetes will increase. Your doctor will check your blood sugar levels to identify if you have gestational diabetes after the twenty-fourth week of pregnancy. If you are at a higher risk, you will need to get tested sooner. Before you go for a gestational diabetes test, you should first drink a drink that is filled with sugar. This will increase the levels of blood sugar in your body. You should take a blood test an hour later to understand how your body has handled the large quantities of sugar. If your test results show that your blood sugar levels are higher than the required cutoff, you will need to conduct more tests. This will mean that you should test the blood sugar when you fast and also take a glucose test after three hours. You may need to take another test later during your pregnancy even if your test results are normal, but you are at a higher risk of developing gestational diabetes.

Gestational Diabetes Treatment

Your doctor will ask you to do the following when you want to treat gestational diabetes:

- Get urine tests done to check the level of ketones in your body
- Always check your levels of blood sugar at least four times a day
- Consume a healthy diet
- Always exercise

Your doctor will constantly track your weight gain, and will also let you know if there is any other medicine that you will need to take to treat gestational diabetes.

Complications of Gestational Diabetes

There are many other complications that can arise because of gestational diabetes.

For The Baby

- Type 2 diabetes later in life
- Early birth
- High birth weight
- Low blood sugar
- Respiratory distress syndrome

For the mother

- Diabetes later in life
- Diabetes in a future pregnancy
- High blood pressure and preeclampsia
- Higher chance of C-section

If you want to prevent gestational diabetes or develop diabetes in the future, you should begin getting yourself tested for diabetes at least eight weeks after you give birth.

Diet & Exercise

Follow the steps mentioned below to prevent gestational diabetes:

- Eat a low-sugar and healthy diet. Ask your nutritionist to develop a meal plan that is prepared for someone who has diabetes. You should switch to natural foods like carrots, raisins and fruit instead of consuming candy, ice cream and cookies. You should also increase your intake of whole grains and vegetables, and watch the size of your servings.

- You should never lose weight during your pregnancy, so if you are overweight try to lose weight before you become pregnant. You should ensure that you are at the ideal weight before you become pregnant.
- Ensure that you always exercise during your pregnancy. If you are trying to conceive, you should begin exercising then. Try to exercise for at least thirty minutes every day.
- You should also ensure that you obtain the appropriate prenatal care. You should take all the necessary tests when you are pregnant, and ensure that you speak to your doctor about your food and your activity.

Chapter Nine

SOME OTHER COMPLICATIONS

*T*here are some other complications that you should be aware of during your pregnancy.

The Activity Level of the Baby Declines

If your baby was previously active, but seems to have less energy now you need not worry. This can be normal, but how will you be able to tell? You can try a few things before you rush to the doctor to understand if there is a problem. Either eat something or drink something cold, and lie on your side. If your baby moves now, you do not have to worry. You should also count the number of times your baby kicks you. You should always set a benchmark of your baby's activity to understand whether your baby is moving less or more. Your baby should kick you at least ten times in two hours, and if he or she kicks lesser number of times, you will need to consult your doctor. Alternatively, you can take an ultrasound to determine the growth and development of the fetus.

. . .

Early Contractions during the Third Trimester

Early contractions are a sign of premature birth. Many first-time mothers cannot differentiate between false labor and true labor. False labor contractions or Braxton-Hicks contractions are non-rhythmic and unpredictable. They also do not increase in intensity. If you drink enough water, these contractions will subside in a few hours. Regular contractions, however, will increase in intensity and they are about ten minutes apart. If you are in your third trimester and you have contractions, you should call the doctor right away. Your doctor can stop the labor if it is too early for your baby to come out.

Water Breaks

You feel water rushing down your legs when you got up from the couch to grab a glass of water. You may think that your water has broken, but it could be urine leakage too. Your bladder is under a lot of pressure during your pregnancy because of the enlarged uterus. It is only for a few women that water breaking will be a dramatic gush of fluid.

You should go to the bathroom immediately and empty your bladder if you are not sure why there is a sudden gush of fluid. If the fluid does not stop, you could have broken your water, and you should go to the hospital.

Flu Symptoms

Experts say that women should always get the flu vaccine during their pregnancy. Women are more likely to get sick during pregnancy, and have some serious complications that are caused by the flu. If you do get the flu, do not rush to the hospital. Talk to your doctor first and see what you can do.

Chapter Ten

EXERCISE AND PREGNANCY

*I*t is important that you perform regular physical activity during your pregnancy since this has multiple benefits. Physical activity will also prepare your body for childbirth. It is important that you understand your body and choose the right exercises to keep you strong. You can modify these exercises to make it easier for you. You do not have to perform strenuous exercises during pregnancy. You must be sensible about the level of exercise that you are performing. You must consult a healthcare professional, doctor, physiotherapist or your midwife to ensure that your exercise routine is not harmful for you or the baby.

Exercise tips

You should never exhaust yourself. Try to perform light exercises during your pregnancy. You will need to reduce the number of exercises you perform and slow down as your pregnancy progresses. If you are ever in doubt, you should consult your doctor or midwife. One way to measure whether the exercise is light or moderate is to see whether you can have a conversation while you exercise. You are probably exercising too much if you are unable to maintain a conversation while you exercise.

If you were never active before you were pregnant, do not take up strenuous exercises immediately. Regardless of the type of exercise you take up, you should let the instructor know that you are pregnant. Make sure that you do not perform more than fifteen minutes of exercise continuously. You can increase the time you spend on exercising to thirty minutes when you feel better. Remember that exercise only should be beneficial and not strenuous.

Some tips that you should keep in mind are:

- Always perform some warm-up and cool-down exercises.
- Try to stay active for at least thirty minutes every day. You can walk for thirty minutes or perform any small exercise for thirty minutes.
- Do not perform any strenuous exercises during humid or hot weather.
- Always drink plenty of water.
- Ensure that your instructor is qualified and is aware that you are pregnant.
- Swimming is a good exercise to consider since the water will support the weight of your fetus.

Exercises to avoid

- After 16 weeks of gestation, you should avoid lying

down on your back since the weight of your bump will press against some blood vessels which will reduce the flow of blood to the fetus and also make you feel weak or faint.

- Avoid any kind of contact sports since there is a risk of you being hit. Do not participate in activities like judo, rugby, football, tennis, squash or kickboxing.
- Avoid downhill skiing, horse riding, cycling, gymnastics and ice hockey since there is a possibility that you may fall.
- Since the fetus does not have any protection from gas embolism or decompression sickness, you should avoid scuba diving.
- You should avoid going to heights above 2,500 meters unless you are acclimatized to the weather conditions in those areas.

Exercises for a fitter pregnancy

You should try to perform the exercises during your pregnancy. These exercises will help to strengthen the muscles in your back and pelvis, allowing you to carry the extra weight. They will also help to improve circulation, make your joints stronger, ease your backache and make you feel better.

#1 Stomach-Strengthening Exercises

When your baby starts growing bigger, you will find that the lower back has a hollow, and this will increase during the pregnancy. This will give you a backache and make it difficult for you to stand. You should perform some abdominal muscle exercises to strength the muscles and ease your backache.

- Lower yourself carefully to the ground and place your hands on your shoulders and knees under the hips.
- Keep your back straight and stretch your fingers forward.
- Take a deep breath in and pull the muscles of your stomach towards your back.
- Now, raise your back up and move your head towards the ceiling. Let your head relax. Ensure that you do not lock your elbows.
- Hold this position for four seconds and move back to the center.
- You must ensure that you do not bend your back. Always keep your back straight. Perform this exercise ten times and make sure that you move the muscles carefully.
- Do not exert yourself or push yourself. Let your back move only as much as it can.

#2 Pelvic Tilt Exercises

- Stand against a wall with your legs shoulder-width apart.
- Slightly bend your knees.
- Breathe in deeply and pull your stomach in towards your spine. Flatten your back against the wall and hold your breath for four seconds. Exhale softly.
- Repeat this exercise ten times.

#3 Pelvic Floor Exercises

Pelvic floor exercises will help to strengthen the muscles on your pelvis. These muscles are under great stress and strain during pregnancy and birth. The pelvis consists of numerous layers of muscles that will stretch to create some support from the end of the backbone to the pubic bone.

Chapter Eleven

TESTS FROM THE LAB

*Y*ou will be asked to take numerous tests, imaging and screenings during your pregnancy, and these tests are designed to help you and the doctor assess the health of your baby. Your doctor will use these tests to optimize the prenatal development and care that you provide to your baby.

Genetic Screening

It is easy to diagnose different types of genetic abnormalities before you give birth to your baby. Your midwife or doctor may ask you to take some genetic tests during your pregnancy if either you or your partner has had a history of different genetic disorders. If you were pregnant with a baby who had a genetic abnormality while still in the womb, it is always a good to take a genetic screening to protect your baby.

· · ·

Some genetic disorders that can be diagnosed before birth are:

- Hemophilia A
- Sickle cell disease
- Cystic fibrosis
- Thalassemia
- Polycystic kidney disease
- Duchenne muscular dystrophy
- Tay-Sachs disease

You can use the screening methods mentioned below during your pregnancy:

- Amniocentesis
- Alpha-fetoprotein (AFP) test or multiple marker test
- Cell-free fetal DNA testing
- Percutaneous umbilical blood sampling (taking a small sample of the baby's blood from the umbilical cord)
- Chorionic villus sampling
- Ultrasound scan

First Trimester Prenatal Tests

During the first trimester, you will need to take a maternal blood test and an ultrasound to check the fetus's development. These tests will help the doctor determine if the fetus is at a risk of developing any birth defects. The screening tests performed during the first trimester include:

1. Ultrasound to determine nuchal translucency: This test will examine the area around the fetus's neck to check for thickening or increased fluid through an ultrasound.

2. Ultrasound to determine the nasal bone: It is difficult to view the nasal bone in some babies who have a chromosome abnormality like Down syndrome. An ultrasound is performed during the eleventh week of gestation to determine the nasal bone.

3. Maternal blood or serum tests: These tests are used to measure the levels of two substances that are found in every pregnant woman:

4. Plasma Protein A: This protein is produced in the first few weeks into pregnancy in the placenta, and abnormal levels of this protein will increase the risk of chromosomal abnormality.

5. Chorionic Gonadotropin: This hormone is also produced in the placenta during the first few weeks into pregnancy, and abnormal levels of this hormone will increase the risk of chromosomal abnormality.

If the results of any of these tests are abnormal, it is important that you seek genetic counseling. Some additional tests like amniocentesis, chorionic villus sampling, ultrasounds and fetal DNA tests will need to be completed to accurately diagnose the issues.

Second Trimester Prenatal Screening Tests

During the second trimester, you will need to take several tests called multiple markers. These tests provide information about any birth defects or genetic disorders that your baby may develop during the pregnancy. These tests are conducted by taking a blood sample between your sixteenth and eighteenth week of pregnancy. Some of these markers include:

1. AFP screening: This test will measure the levels of the serum AFP in your blood during your pregnancy. AFP is a protein that is produced by the amniotic fluid that covers the fetus, and this protein can enter your blood when it passes through the placenta. If your blood has abnormal levels of AFP, it can indicate the following:
2. Defects in the wall of the abdomen in the fetus
3. Since the levels are different throughout the pregnancy, it can indicate a miscalculated due date
4. Chromosomal abnormalities like Down syndrome
5. Spina bifida and other neural tube defects
6. Twins – in this instance, the higher levels of AFP in your blood are because two fetuses are producing the same protein
7. Estriol, inhibin and chorionic gonadotropin are hormones that can be used to determine the health of the fetus. This hormone is produced in the placenta.

Any abnormal results in these tests mean that some additional testing will need to be done to eliminate doubt. Your doctor may ask you to take an ultrasound to check the health of the fetus and also reassess the milestones of your pregnancy. When you have performed the tests during your first and second trimester, you can use the results to confirm whether your fetus is healthy or not.

. . .

Ultrasound

An ultrasound scan is used to create an image of the baby and the internal organs using high-frequency sound waves. An ultrasound is performed during your pregnancy to verify the due date and check the growth of the fetus.

When Is An Ultrasound Performed During Pregnancy?

An ultrasound is performed during the pregnancy for numerous reasons:

First Trimester

- Detect any abnormalities in the fetus
- Examine the anatomy of the uterus
- Determine the number of fetuses
- Assess the due date
- Diagnose miscarriage or ectopic pregnancy

Mid-trimester

- Reassess the due date if necessary
- Assist in some prenatal tests
- Examine the fetus for abnormalities if any
- Check the quantity of amniotic fluid
- Monitor the growth of the fetus
- Examine the flow of blood
- Observe fetal activity and behavior
- Measure the length of the cervix

Third Trimester

- Monitor the growth of the fetus
- Check the quantity of amniotic fluid
- Assess the placenta
- Determine the position of the fetus
- Conduct a biophysical profile test

CONCLUSION

Thank you for purchasing the book.

Pregnancy is one of the most exciting times of a woman's life, but it is also one of the most sensitive periods of her life. A woman will need to take numerous things into account with respect to her nutrition to ensure that she and her baby are safe. Over the course of this book, you will gather information on different supplements you can take to prevent deficiencies and different complications during pregnancy. I hope you gather all the information you are looking for and are healthy during your pregnancy.

SOURCES

https://www.webmd.com/baby/features/7-pregnancy-warning-signs#2

https://www.pregnancybirthbaby.org.au/search-results/complications

https://www.healthline.com/health/pregnancy/delivery-complications#risk-factors

https://www.pregnancybirthbaby.org.au/pregnancy-complications

https://www.pregnancybirthbaby.org.au/severe-vomiting-during-pregnancy-hyperemesis-gravidarum

https://www.pregnancybirthbaby.org.au/bleeding-during-pregnancy

https://www.pregnancybirthbaby.org.au/itching-during-pregnancy

https://www.pregnancybirthbaby.org.au/pre-eclampsia

https://www.healthline.com/nutrition/supplements-during-pregnancy#TOC_TITLE_HDR_5

https://www.healthline.com/health/high-blood-pressure-hypertension/during-pregnancy#complications

https://www.webmd.com/diabetes/gestational-diabetes#2

https://www.pregnancybirthbaby.org.au/exercising-during-pregnancy

https://www.hopkinsmedicine.org/health/wellness-and-prevention/common-tests-during-pregnancy

FOOD FOR PREGNANCY VOLUME 3

The Mom's Guide to Understanding the Best
Supplements and Nutrients for a Healthy Growing Baby

INTRODUCTION

I want to thank you for choosing the book, *'Food for Pregnancy Volume 3 - The Moms Guide to Understanding the Best Supplements and Nutrients for a Healthy Growing Baby'*

The first two volumes of the book provided information on the different types of food that you are allowed to eat. Those volumes helped you understand why it was important for you to watch your diet during your pregnancy. This book will discuss something a little more important.

You are bound to be under immense stress during pregnancy, and this will lead to some issues during labor or after pregnancy. It is extremely important that you understand how to deal with this stress. This book sheds some light on why women may be under undue stress during pregnancy, and also provides some tips that you can use to overcome that stress. You will also gather information about some toxins that you should be wary of, and what you should do to avoid any exposure to those toxins.

You have taken care of yourself and have given birth to a healthy new baby. Now, what do you do? How do you care for your body? This book will shed some light on the different changes you can expect in your body, and also talks about how you can handle those changes. I hope the information in this book will help you go through pregnancy with ease.

Chapter One

TOXINS TO AVOID DURING PREGNANCY

*W*hen you are pregnant, you are advised to avoid alcohol and to stop smoking. Research shows that consumption of alcohol during pregnancy can lead to fetal alcohol syndrome, and smoking increases the risk of stillbirth, sudden infant death syndrome and miscarriage. It does seem a bit strange when people ask you to give up on using nail polish, using air freshener or drinking water from plastic bottles doesn't it? Research conducted by the Environmental Working Group (EWG) shows that the chemicals in these products are not safe for you or your baby, and they can be as toxic as alcohol or smoke. The chemicals present in these products will get into your blood stream and will pass to the fetus through the placenta. If these toxins are passed through to the fetus during the developmental stages, it can cause irreversible or permanent organ and brain damage. This damage will not just be present at birth but will continue into adulthood.

The research conducted by EWG concluded that a baby could be born with close to 232 industrial pollutants and compounds. Some of these pollutants and compounds are found in water and soil, and it is impossible to avoid them. There are others that can be found in house paint and shampoos, and it is easy to avoid these. This chapter lists ten pollutants that you should protect yourself and your baby from.

Lead

Lead is a powerful neurotoxic metal known to cause nervous system disorders, permanent brain damage, hyperactivity and learning and behavior difficulties. If you are exposed to this metal during your pregnancy, you may endanger your child. Lead is known to slow down the growth of a child, both in the uterus and after their birth.

How do you think exposure occurs? You may drink water from the tap, and this water may be contaminated with lead. Lead contaminates water if the pipes are maintained poorly or the metal is very old. This is what happened in a city in Michigan. You may also inhale some dust tainted with lead from chipping or old paint. You could be working in a garden where the soil is contaminated by lead because of a building that was last painted in the year 1978. Lead was banned from paints only after 1978. There are some lipsticks that have some lead in them because the pigments used to give the lipstick some color contain lead.

How to Avoid Lead

You should ensure that the tap that you use for water is free of lead. You should check the Consumer Confidence Report issued by the water utility in your area. If the tap water not free of lead, you should contact the officials in your area and demand that they repair the water system in the area. Alternatively, you can purchase a filter that will filter any contaminants, including lead, from the water.

If your house was built before the year 1978, you should use a test kit and verify if the paint is free of lead or not. The results of your test will tell you if you need to call a lead-abatement specialist. If you want to renovate an older home, you should vacate the residence and move to a lead-free area. If you do want to use cosmetics, you should stick to using organic products where the pigments used are natural fruit pigments.

Mercury

Mercury is another neurotoxic that will impede the development of the brain and nervous system. The mercury that we are exposed to is through air pollution. When a power plant burns coal, it releases mercury into the air, which then falls into fresh water lakes, rivers, streams and oceans. It will then accumulate in fish like shark, tilefish, king mackerel, swordfish and tuna. Mercury is also present in older thermometers and fluorescent light bulbs, but the highest exposure comes through seafood that has mercury in it.

How to Avoid Mercury

As mentioned in the previous books, you should consume seafood that is low in mercury, but rich in omega-3 fatty acids, like tilapia, anchovies, shrimp, cod, pollock, trout and sardines. You should also switch to using a digital thermometer or use a CFL bulb or LED bulb, as these are energy efficient.

PCBs

PCBs or polychlorinated bisphenols were labeled as possible human carcinogens by the U. S. Environmental Protection Agency (EPA). PCBs also damage the human immune, neurological and reproductive systems. These compounds have been banned since the year 1976, but they can still be found in animals and people who live near areas where PCBs used to be produced.

People often ingest PCBs through food. As mentioned earlier, soil may get contaminated because of PCBs. Cattle that graze on this soil will be contaminated with PCBs. Studies conducted by researchers in the state of Washington found that there were high levels of PCBs in the packaging of some foods like macaroni and cheese, taco shells, cheese and cracker snack packs and more. PCBs are also used in inks and coloring, and have been found in magazines, house paints and newspapers.

How to Avoid PCBs

Studies show that PCBs are found in large quantities in fat, and it is for this reason that you should avoid consuming fatty fish and red meat. You should always trim the fat from any of the foods that you eat. It is a good idea to consume grains, organic fruit and vegetables instead of consuming processed food. You should also switch to non-toxic primers and paints.

Formaldehyde

Formaldehyde is a pollutant that is found in most products, especially household products like cabinets, furniture made from pressed wood, chairs, couches and other furniture, fabric softeners and carpeting. This pollutant is also used in shampoos, nail polishes and cosmetics as a preservative.

People are often exposed to formaldehyde when the chemical evaporates from the product it is in and mixes with the air. Studies show that formaldehyde has negative effects on the immune system. Studies conducted on lab animals showed that formaldehyde will lead to low birth weight.

How to Avoid Formaldehyde

It is important that you read the labels carefully and only purchase those products that are free of formaldehyde. If you do want to use nail polish, you should choose those products that are free of formaldehyde and other chemicals. Make sure that you always paint your nails in a well-ventilated room. If you are installing cabinets or carpets in your house, make sure that you leave your windows open.

Always purchase cabinets that are made fully of wood instead of purchasing products that are made using particle-boards or pressed wood. Do not use air fresheners with aerosol, atomized perfume and plug-in fragrance dispensers.

Phthalates

Plastic is often softened using a chemical compound called a phthalate. These chemicals make it easy for companies to make smooth body lotion, prevent the hair spray from getting stiff and also make nail polish easy to apply. If you use capsules, there is a possibility that you may consume phthalates. These chemicals are also used to deliver fragrances. They are used in household cleaning products, perfumes, commercial air fresheners, personal care products and detergents to release their smells.

Studies were conducted on male lab animals to understand the effects of phthalates on males. These studies concluded that phthalates can lead to decreased sperm count, infertility, malformations of the urethra and penis and unde-scended testes. Studies conducted by the National Institutes of Health concluded that phthalates reduced the chances of pregnancy in women, and these studies also showed that children who were born to women who were exposed to phthalates during their pregnancy were at a higher risk of developing ADHD. These babies may also be born with a low birth weight, may be born prematurely or may be susceptible to becoming overweight later in life.

How to Avoid Phthalates

Make sure you always read labels. You should always substitute the air fresheners that are made with synthetic fragrances, including plug-in air fresheners, hanging car air fresheners, air sprays with fragrances with phthalate-free products. You should always use fewer personal care products since your skin absorbs the chemicals from the different products you use. You should avoid microwaving any food in a plastic container since the phthalates from the plastic will move into the food. You should also avoid using vinyl rain-coats and shower curtains since vinyl also contains phthalates.

Flame Retardants

Polybrominated diphenyl ethers or PBDEs are industrial chemicals used to retard flames especially in furniture, plastic and mattresses. These chemicals can be exposed to the air, soil and water when they are used and manufactured. They are not water soluble, and they tend to settle at the bottom of lakes or rivers, and as a result can accumulate in fish. These chemicals also mix with the house dust. PBDEs will interfere with the metabolism, development of the brain and nervous system and growth. It is for this reason that children who are affected by PBDEs have lower cognitive abilities. PBDEs also contribute to some disease in adults.

How to Avoid PBDEs

PBDEs are used to manufacture foam and upholstery. If you have any old furniture at home, there are chances that the stuffing or the cushion is being exposed. You will need to either cover this or replace the decor to reduce the concentration of PBDEs in the dust. You can also purchase furniture free of PBDEs. Make sure that you choose any electronic made with alternatives to flame-retardants.

Toluene

Toluene is a colorless and a clear liquid with a distinctive smell. This chemical is a good solvent and is used in paint thinners, paints, lacquers, nail polish, rubber, printing, leather tanning processes and adhesives. This chemical is also added to gasoline along with xylene and benzene to improve the ratings of octane. Toluene is often present in the air when there is a lot of traffic. This chemical easily evaporates and is a source of air pollution. If you leave paint or nail polish open for too long, the toluene in the products will evaporate into the air.

Women who are exposed to high levels of toluene during pregnancy are at a higher risk. Toluene can also affect the functions of the liver and kidney, harm the reproductive system and also reduce immunity towards specific diseases. You should ensure that you do not expose yourself to large quantities of toluene.

How to Avoid Toluene

You should always ensure that you purchase those nail polishes that do not have toluene and formaldehyde. You should never refinish or repaint your furniture or refinish your cupboards or banisters when you are pregnant. If you do want to repaint your house, you should use water-based paints. Do not use any paints that you will need to wash off using a paint thinner. If you are filling your car up with gas, make sure that you walk away so you do not inhale the fumes.

PFOS or PFOA

PFOA and PFOS are chemicals that are formulated to produce or manufacture stick and stain resistant. These chemicals are organic compounds that are pre-fluorinated. These compounds are used in fast-food containers, carpeting and furniture, non-stick cooking pans and pots, microwave popcorn bags, pizza boxes and stain resistant clothing. Exposure to pre-fluorinated organic compounds increases the risk of low birth weight. Research is still being conducted to understand the impact that these compounds have on the fetus.

Research conducted in the John Hopkins Bloomberg School of Public Health concluded that pregnant women who had elevated levels of these compounds in their birth gave birth to children who had low weights. These babies also had a smaller head circumference when compared to those babies who were born to women who were not exposed to these chemicals. These conditions led to some medical problems in children later in their lives. Other studies have shown that exposure to these chemicals leads to elevated cholesterol levels, difficulty in conceiving and low sperm quality.

How To Avoid PFOA or PFOS

You should always avoid stain-resistant furniture and ensure that you do not use any stain protection products on your furniture or carpets. You should avoid wearing stain-resistant clothing, and only purchase those clothes that you can launder easily. Make sure that you use napkins when you eat, and never leave any non-stick pots or pans on the gas stove unattended. Never place these pots or pans on high temperatures. If the pans start to deteriorate, you should either get rid of them or replace them with new pots and pans. Try to use seasoned cast iron or stainless-steel cookware.

Asbestos

The compound asbestos is a combination of six fibrous minerals, and research shows that these minerals cause cancer. This material can resist fire, and it is for this reason that this material is used in most parts of the home, including vinyl flooring, attic and pipe insulation, roofing shingles, ceiling tiles, clothing, sheetrock and automotive products like drum brake linings and disc brake pads. The asbestos fibers will be exposed to the air when the products become old, which makes it easy to inhale the chemical. Asbestos is also known to contaminate water because it is found in some rocks and in soil. There are some pre-mixed potting and garden soils that may also have some content of asbestos in them. There is no safe level of exposure to this chemical.

How to Avoid Asbestos

When you are checking the quality of water in your area, make sure that you also check for any asbestos content in the water. Water suppliers are required to adhere the Safe Drinking Water Act, which states that they will need to remove asbestos from water fully. If it is difficult for them to remove asbestos completely, they should bring the concentration down to 1 MFL. If you see that the report shows that there is a higher concentration, you should meet your city or county representative, and ask them to look into the matter. You should use filters that will help to remove both asbestos and lead from the water.

If you live in a house that was built before the year 1980, you should remember that some of the construction components might be contaminated. You should hire an expert to sample the products in the house and determine the concentration of asbestos. These experts can determine if the items should be removed or if the asbestos can be contained in one place alone. Alternatively, you should hire a certified professional who can clean up the asbestos content in the house. If you love gardening, you should not use vermiculite to improve the quality of the potting soil. You should try to use sawdust, peat, bark or perlite.

Bisphenol A or BPA

Hard polycarbonate plastic used to make bottles, jugs, tableware like cups and plates, food storage containers and baby bottles is made using the petrochemical Bisphenol A or BPA. This compound is also used in thermal cash register receipts and epoxy resin, which is used to line beverage and food cans to prevent any bacterial contamination and corrosion. BPA is a very functional compound, but it is a highly unstable chemical. This compound will leach into the liquids and food from the packaging.

BPA can disrupt the endocrine system in the body, even if it is consumed in small doses. Any exposure to BPA is harmful to the fetus since it can disrupt the development. This chemical increases the risk of developing prostate and breast cancer, changes in gender specific behavior due to changes in brain development and the early onset of puberty. This chemical is also linked to infertility, heart disease, toddler behavior problems, diabetes, erectile dysfunction and miscarriages.

How to Avoid BPA

If you want to decrease your exposure to BPA, you should reduce the number of plastic water bottles you use. You should avoid using the bottles that are labeled as BPA-free. Use aluminum, stainless steel or glass bottles instead. Avoid consuming canned foods and drinks and choose fresh or frozen juices and foods. Instead of consuming carbonated drinks, you should try to drink juices or water out of glass bowls. If you want to eat beans, make sure that you do not buy canned beans. Always soak the beans overnight and cook them before you eat them.

It is difficult to know if a receipt has some BPA in it. So, leave the receipt behind if you are sure that you do not need it. Alternatively, ask the store to email the receipt to you. When you are at the grocery store, you can ask the cashier to drop the receipt in the bag. Remember to never place the receipt in your mouth.

Chapter Two

STRESS AND PREGNANCY

ou will notice that your body and your emotions will change during your pregnancy. You will also notice that your life is changing, and so are the lives of every member in your family. You will welcome these changes with happiness, but it is important that you know that these changes will add new stress to your life.

It is common for you to be under a lot of stress during pregnancy. That said, too much stress will make it hard for you to be happy during your pregnancy. You will have headaches, overeat, lose your appetite or even have trouble sleeping.

If you are under high stress for long periods, it will lead to some health problems like high blood pressure and also increase the risk of developing some heart issues. If you are suffering under high stress, you may also give birth earlier than the scheduled date. The chances of low birth weight also increase. If your baby is born too soon or is too small, they are at a higher risk of developing some health problems.

. . .

Causes of Stress during Pregnancy

There are different reasons why women are under stress during pregnancy, but there are a few common reasons:

- You may have a backache, nausea, and constipation or feel tired due to pregnancy; it is normal for women to face these discomforts during pregnancy.
- Your mood is bound to change because your hormones keep fluctuating. It becomes very hard for you to handle stress when your mood constantly changes.
- You are probably worried about what can happen during labor or may be worried about how you will care for your child after you give birth.
- If you are working, you are under a lot of pressure to manage your responsibilities and also prepare your colleagues so they can manage your work when you are away from your job.
- It is true that your life may take some unexpected turns, and this is not going to stop because you are pregnant. The changes in your life will affect you and may sometimes cause undue stress.

Types of Stress that Cause Problems during Pregnancy

Every woman is under stress during pregnancy, and if you handle this stress well, you can take on many other challenges. Regular stress like sitting in traffic and work deadlines will not lead to any problems during pregnancy. That said, if you are under undue stress during your pregnancy, the risk of problems like premature birth will increase. Women who are

under stress during pregnancy can give birth to healthy
babies, but you will need to be careful if you experience the
following kinds of stress:

- ***Negative Life Events***

You will be under stress if you lose a job or home or are going
through a divorce, some illness or have witnessed a death in
the family. These events will lead to immense stress, which
can harm you and your baby.

- ***Catastrophic Events***

Events like terrorist attacks, earthquakes and hurricanes
also lead to undue stress.

- ***Long-lasting Stress***

Long-lasting stress is caused when you are being abused at
home or at work, are depressed, are having serious health
problems or are facing some financial problems. If you are
suffering from depression, you will be upset and sad for long
periods making it hard for you to lead a normal life.

- ***Racism***

Quite a few women face stress caused due to racism. It is
for this reason that African-American women are at a higher
risk of giving birth to babies with low birth weight or may
give birth to babies before the schedules date when compared
to women from other ethnic or racial groups.

- ***Pregnancy Related Stress***

Women are always under stress during their pregnancy, and they add to this stress by constantly worrying about the health of their baby, whether they can handle the pain during labor, how they will be as a parent and about losing their baby. If you find yourself thinking this way, you should speak to your doctor or midwife.

Post-Traumatic Stress Disorder (PTSD) and Pregnancy

PTSD or Post-Traumatic Stress Disorder is when you have trouble after you experience or witness a terrible event like abuse, the loss of a loved one, a natural disaster, a terrorist attack or rape. People who have PTSD may have the following when they are reminded of the event:

- Nightmares
- Flashbacks of the event
- Serious anxiety
- Physical responses like sweating, racing heartbeat and nausea

Almost eight percent of women suffer from PTSD during their pregnancy, and they are likely to give birth to babies with low birth weight or may give birth before the scheduled date when compared to women who do not have PTSD. Women suffering from PTSD commonly smoke cigarettes, take street drugs or drink alcohol to cope with the anxiety or fear caused due to PTSD. When they behave in this manner, they may have many problems during their pregnancy. If you suffer from PTSD, it is important that you speak to your doctor or midwife and get into contact with a mental health professional who can guide you.

. . .

Does stress cause problems during a pregnancy?

Most people do not understand what the effects of stress are on pregnancy. There are some stress-related hormones that can cause numerous complications in pregnancy. Long-lasting stress or serious stress can affect your immune system, and this will increase the chances of developing an infection. Since your immune system is weak, there are chances that you may develop some uterine infections that can lead to premature birth.

Stress will also affect the way you respond to some situations in life. You may start to consume alcohol, or start smoking and may resort to taking street drugs to endure that stress which can lead to some problems in your pregnancy.

How does stress affect your baby later in life?

It is known that high levels of stress can lead to some problems during pregnancy and even after you give birth. Stress affects the development of your child's brain and immune system, and as a result your child may find it hard to pay attention or may be anxious at all times.

Chapter Three

HOW TO DEAL WITH STRESS DURING PREGNANCY?

$\mathcal{A}$s mentioned earlier, you are bound to be slightly stressed about the numerous changes that are taking place in your body during your pregnancy. If you are only stressed occasionally, you will not have any trouble with your pregnancy. If you are anxious, irritable and stressed throughout the day and for long periods, you should speak to your doctor or midwife to understand why you feel this way. Prolonged or extreme stress can increase the risk of low birth weight. You may not be affected too badly because of the stress that you are under, but it is important that you tackle your issues now so you can enjoy the joys that pregnancy brings.

How to Reduce Stress

Let us look at ten steps that you can take to reduce stress during your pregnancy.

#1 Always Focus On Your Baby

It is important that you take some time out of your busy schedule and focus on yourself. Studies show that it is important for both you and your baby that you relax, so you should never worry about taking some time for yourself. If you have read the books, you know that your baby can hear your voice from the 23rd week, so you should try to sing, read or chat with your baby bump. This is one of the best ways to bond with your child, and you will feel much better about your pregnancy.

#2 Sleep Well

You should always listen to your body. Make sure that you take a nap or go to bed early if you feel too tired. It is also okay to take a break from work if you are tired. Studies show that sleep is important for mental health, and if you are happy, you will have a healthy pregnancy. There are numerous tips that you can use to make sure that you sleep well during your pregnancy.

- Develop a sleep schedule, and make sure that you stick to it. Wake up and go to bed at the same time every day. It is true that you may want to sleep in on some days but remember that when you do that it will be harder for you to sleep at night.
- Get a relaxing massage before bed.
- Create a soothing ritual for yourself before you go to bed. Take a relaxing bath, read a good book or have a warm drink before you get ready for bed.

It is very hard for you to get the rest you need when you become a parent. You still deserve to take some rest. You can always ask your partner, parents, grandparents or friends to look after your child for a few hours so you can have some rest. Take a break for yourself and spend the time doing something you love to do.

#3 *Talk about It*

If you have any personal problem or are worried about the wellbeing of your baby, you should always talk about it. Speak to your doctor or your midwife about what you are feeling. You should never be afraid of how you truly feel. It is only when you are honest about how you feel that you can get all the support. Your doctor and midwife will have seen so many women go through similar issues and would love to help you overcome your fears instead of letting you suffer in silence. You can also talk to your partner. You may find that your partner is also worried and has some other concerns. It is only when you talk things through that you will feel better about the situation.

If it makes you feel better, you can speak to other pregnant women during an exercise class or a doctor's visit. They may also have the same feelings as you and will want to hear you out.

#4 *Eat Well*

It is important that you eat well and eat the right food. The food you eat will provide nourishment for your body, your brain and your baby. The first two volumes of the series provided information about the different types of foods you can and cannot eat. You should ensure that you eat meals at regular intervals to ensure that your blood sugar levels do not drop. When your blood sugar levels drop, you will be more irritable and tired.

It is not easy for you to eat well if you do not feel too good about it. If you suffer from morning sickness or nausea, you will avoid food. But you should find a way to consume at least one full meal every day. This will make you feel better. You should also ensure that you drink at least eight glasses of water every day. If you do not consume enough water, you will be dehydrated, and this will affect your mood.

Before you were pregnant, you may have had a glass of wine to help you unwind, but you should avoid alcohol when you are pregnant. You can drink a warm glass of milk instead of wine.

#5 *Try Exercise*

You may not want to exercise, and this is probably the last thing that will cross your mind, especially when you are pregnant. However, exercise is known to lift a person's spirits at any time. One of the reasons why doctors advise people to exercise is that it helps to release the chemical dopamine in your brain. This chemical is a feel-good chemical. You can do different types of exercises during your pregnancy, and these have been listed in the second volume of the series. You should ensure that you speak to your doctor or midwife before you join any activity. One of the best exercises to do during your pregnancy is swimming. This activity will keep your body toned and will not be too hard on your joints.

You can also join a class for pregnancy yoga. Yoga not only stretches the muscles in your body, but also helps you learn a few meditation techniques that you can use to relax and calm your mind. These techniques will boost your emotional well-being. It is a good idea to add a few minutes of exercise to your daily schedule. You can walk around the house as often as you can for ten minutes. If you love being outdoors, you can take a walk in the park.

#6 *Prepare For Birth*

It is important that you understand what can happen during labor. You should sign up for some classes to understand this better. When you know what you can expect and understand all your options, you will feel confident. It is also a good idea to speak to your doctor or midwife to understand what you can expect from pregnancy, and also ask as many questions as you can. Your doctor or midwife can help you write a plan that will help you define your preferences. There is no harm with making changes to your plan later. It is important that you keep the plan flexible. This will help you remain calm even if the birth does not happen the way you imagined it to.

If you are giving birth in a birth center or a hospital, you can ask your doctor to let you visit the delivery room beforehand. When you are familiar with your surroundings, you will feel better about the whole process and this will help you set your mind to rest. If you are terrified of giving birth and would prefer to have caesarean, you should speak to your doctor or midwife. They can help you handle the fear and anxiety, and also refer you to a therapist who can help you work through your issues. You will feel better about giving birth at the end.

#7 Cope With Commuting

One of the major sources of stress is travel, and this will become worse when you are heavily pregnant. It is unfortunate that your employer only has to worry about work related travel. He is not obligated to think about how you commute to work daily. Having said that, some employers make the effort to help you through your pregnancy and change the shift timings for you, so you do not have to work odd hours or commute during traffic.

It is important for you to keep track of how you sit on

public transport. If nobody offers to give you a seat, you can request them to give you one. Pregnant women are given first-class tickets on some trains. You can visit the operator's website to learn more about these tickets.

#8 Sort Out Any Money Issues

Most women worry about how they are going to pay for the equipment and clothes that they need once they give birth. If you are worried, just sit down and make a list of everything you need. You can also see if there are some items that you can borrow from your family or friends.

You do not have to buy everything on your list. You will need baskets and cribs only for a short duration, and you can borrow these items from your friends. You can also buy many of the items second-hand. If you do not want to buy these products online, you can ask a friend to help you out.

If you are constantly worried about money and about how you are going to give your baby a good start, you should speak to your doctor or midwife. You can also get in touch with the local children's center to see where you can get some of the items that you are looking for. You can check with your employer if you are eligible for any programs at work and see if there are any benefits that you can claim. It is important that you ensure that you get your full maternity leave and pay. Speak to your human resources manager and understand the different benefits and support that your employer is offering.

#9 Attend Complementary Therapies

One of the best ways to de-stress is to take a massage. You can ask your partner to give you a lower back massage, and if they do not know how to do it show them a video to help them understand the same. You can also ask them to give you a relaxation massage. If you do not want their help, you can learn how you can give yourself a foot massage. Many beauty salons and spas provide different pregnancy massage treatments. You must ensure that the person giving you the massage is qualified to work with pregnant women. Some studies show that aromatherapy helps to reduce anxiety. It also helps you feel relaxed and calm.

#10 Be Mindful

Mindfulness is one of the best ways to connect with your surroundings. You can enjoy every moment, and not think about negative things. This means that you will need to spend all your energy and focus only on those moments in life where you are ecstatic, like when you first felt your baby kick. Research shows that practicing mindfulness helps to ease worry, depression, stress and anxiety in pregnant women. Let us look at some tips you can use to be mindful every day in your life:

- Always pay attention to the scents, sounds, sights and any other sensation around you when you are going about your day. It will be hard to do this at all times, so take some time out every day and focus on everything that you are experiencing.
- If you have the same routine every day, you can stop and look at the familiar things around you. You should always try to do something new every day, like take a different route, walk to a different shop or sit in a different place every time you step out for a walk.
- Always take some time out to focus on your thoughts and pay attention to the flow of your thoughts. Let your mind drift and see how your

thoughts flow. Make sure that you give each thought or feeling a name and try to identify some pattern between those thoughts and feelings.

- You can also practice mindfulness meditation. You will need to close your eyes and focus only on your breathing or the sounds around you. If you find your mind wandering, you should bring it back.

#11 Treat Yourself

One of the best ways to relax is to laugh. Try to read a good novel, watch some funny videos or movies, play funny games with your partner or meet up with your friends. You should spend on all the beauty treatments during your pregnancy.

What If You Are Still Stressed?

You should speak to your doctor or midwife if your stress levels are too high. The minute you start to feel overwhelmed, you should meet your doctor. You could be suffering either from depression or anxiety, or you may need some help to stop thinking negatively. We all need someone to help us sort our thoughts out.

Your doctor or midwife may ask you to attend some support group meetings or may refer you to a psychotherapist or counselor. You may also be asked to undergo cognitive behavior therapy depending on the severity of your stress. Your doctor or midwife may give you some strategies that you can use to help you tackle the anxiety or depression.

If you are taking any medication for any mental health condition like depression, you must ensure that you do not stop taking it abruptly. Ask your doctor what the risks of taking this medication are during your pregnancy. You may need to continue to take the medication or may be asked to undergo cognitive behavior therapy.

You may feel that your stress is not too bad, and that you are not anxious or depression. If it still bothers you, you should speak to your doctor or midwife during any of your appointments. When you get the right help, you can cope with stress during pregnancy and even after you give birth.

Chapter Four

YOUR BODY AFTER PREGNANCY

*a*s mentioned earlier, your body goes through many changes when you give birth, and these changes can be both emotional and physical. It is important for you to learn more about any postpartum discomforts that you may have after birth and see what you can do to overcome that discomfort. Before you treat any discomfort that you may be feeling, you should speak to your doctor or midwife. There are some medicines that you should not take when you are breastfeeding. Make sure that you attend all your checkups even if you do not feel any different. There are some conditions that will need to be treated immediately after you give birth.

Changes in Your Body A Few Weeks after You Give Birth

Your body will go through many changes after you have a baby. You will notice that your body went through numerous changes during pregnancy, and your body worked very hard to keep you and your baby healthy and safe. Your body will change again after you give birth. Some of the changes that your body goes through are physical, like your breasts growing larger and being full of milk, while others are emotional, like stress.

It is normal to be slightly uncomfortable after you give birth, and it is normal for your body to change. That said, some of the changes and discomfort that you feel could be symptoms of health issues, and you should treat these changes immediately. Ensure that you go for all your checkups even if you think you are okay. It is important to visit the doctor regularly after you give birth to ensure that you are recovering well. Your doctor can spot any irregularities and inform you immediately. It is important that you take care of yourself since new mothers are at a higher risk of developing some life-threatening complications a few weeks after they give birth.

What is perineum soreness?

The area between your rectum and vagina is called the perineum. This area will stretch, and may tear, during labor and birth. This area is often very sore after you give birth and could be sorer if you choose to have an episiotomy. An episiotomy is a cut made in the perineum to help the baby come out. If you do feel sore, you can try the following:

- Perform some Kegel exercises. Kegel exercises will strengthen the muscles in the pelvic area. When you do this exercise, you should squeeze the muscles in your pelvic region that you use to stop yourself from passing urine. You should hold these muscles tight for at least ten seconds and release them. Repeat this exercise ten times and perform the exercise at least thrice a day.

- Place a cold pack on the perineum. You can either buy a cold pack and place it in your freezer or wrap ice in a towel and use it as a cold pack.
- Always sit on a donut-shaped pillow or cushion.
- Always take a warm bath.
- You may develop infections while the episiotomy is healing. Make sure that you wipe your pelvic region after you go to the bathroom to prevent the development of any infection.
- Speak to your doctor to understand how you can deal with the soreness.

What are afterbirth pains?

Your uterus would have expanded during pregnancy to provide enough space to your baby, and it will need to shrink to its regular size once you give birth. When your uterus is shrinking, you will feel some cramps in your belly. These cramps will go away in a few days. When you are pregnant, your uterus will weigh close to 2.5 ounces, and is hard and round. When your uterus shrinks back to its size, it will only weigh two ounces. If the pain is unbearable, you can ask your doctor to prescribe some medication to ease the pain.

Changes in the Body after a Cesarean

If you choose to give birth through a C-section or cesarean, your doctor will make a cut in your uterus and belly to help the baby come out. This is a major surgery, and your body will take some time to recover. You may be extremely tired during the first few days after you give birth because you may have lost a lot of blood during the procedure. The cut on your belly will be sore. Here are some tips to help you deal with the pain and the changes:

- If you feel a lot of pain, you can ask the doctor to provide you with some pain medication. Never take a medicine without checking with your doctor.
- Since you will be tired, you should ask your partners, friends or family to help you with the baby.
- Try to get enough rest. Make sure that you sleep when your baby sleeps. This means that you should sleep during the day too.
- Never lift any object that is heavier than your baby.
- Do not squat.
- Always support your belly when you are feeding your baby.
- Replace the fluids in your body by drinking enough water.

Vaginal Discharge

Your body will need to get rid of all the tissue and blood that was present inside your uterus to protect your baby. It will need to remove these from the body, and this discharge is called lochia or vaginal discharge. You will see that the discharge is bright red and can have some blood clots in it. This will only happen for a few days after you give birth. Over time, the flow will reduce, and the discharge will become lighter. You may have this discharge for a few weeks or a month. You will need to wear sanitary pads until the flow stops.

. . .

Breast Engorgement

A few weeks after you give birth, your breasts will begin to fill with milk. They will feel very sore and tender, but this discomfort will go away quickly when you start feeding your baby regularly. If you do not want to breastfeed, the tenderness will last until your breasts will stop making milk. This will happen in a few days. You can use the tips below to help you during this phase:

- Always feed your baby. Never take a long break between feedings and do not miss a feeding. You must never skip feeding your baby in the night.
- You should always remove some milk from your breasts before you feed your baby. You can do this by pressing your breasts with your hand or through a breast pump.
- Always lay on warm towels or take a warm shower to help the milk flow. If your breasts are very tender, you should use cold packs.
- When you are not feeding, your breasts may lead. To prevent your clothes from getting wet, you should wear nursing pads in your bra.
- If your breasts are painful and are still swollen, you should speak to your doctor to understand why.
- If you do not want to breastfeed, you should wear a supportive and firm bra.

Nipple Pain

You may feel some pain around your nipples when you breastfeed. You will feel this pain during the first few days, and the pain worsens if your nipples begin to crack. Let us look at some tips to help you handle the pain:

- Speak to a lactation consultant or your doctor and ensure that your baby is sucking on your nipples in the right way.
- Ask your doctor to prescribe some cream that you can use on your nipples.
- After you are done feeding, massage your nipples and breasts with some milk, and do not cover your breasts until they are dry.

Swelling

Many women will have some swelling in their face, hand and feet during pregnancy, and this is caused due to the accumulation of the excess fluid in your body. It will take time for this swelling to reduce even after you give birth. Use the following tips to help you with easing the swelling:

- Always lie on your left side when you are sleeping or resting.
- Pull your feet up and sit.
- Make sure that you wear loose clothes and always stay cool.
- Drink a lot of water.

Hemorrhoids

The veins around the anus can begin to pain or may be swollen. These veins are called hemorrhoids, and they may bleed or hurt after you give birth. It is common to have hemorrhoids during pregnancy and after you give birth. Let us look at some tips that will help you deal with hemorrhoids:

- Always take a warm water bath.
- Speak to your doctor and see if you can use a cream or spray to ease the pain.
- Consume foods like whole-grain cereals or bread, vegetables and fruit to increase your fiber intake.
- Drink a lot of water.
- Never strain yourself too much when you are pooping.

Constipation

There are times when you find it difficult to pass stools because you do not have any bowel movements. This is called constipation. You will find that you are constipated for a few days after giving birth. If you have constipation, use the following tips:

- Always consume foods that are rich in fiber.
- Drink a lot of fluids.
- Speak to your provider to understand what medicine you can take to ease the constipation.

Urinary Problems after Giving Birth

You may have a burning sensation or feel pain when you urinate after you give birth. There may be times when you want to urinate, but you are unable to while there will be times when you want to stop urinating, but you cannot. This condition is called incontinence and it will go away when

your muscles in the pelvic region become strong again. If you
are having trouble with urinating, use the tips given below:

- Drink plenty of water.
- Always leave a tap running when you want to go to
  the bathroom.
- Take a warm bath.
- Speak to your provider if the pain continues.

Sweating After Giving Birth

You may sweat too much at night after you give birth, and
this is caused because the hormones in your body are changing. Wear loose clothes when you go to bed and try to avoid
covering yourself with too many blankets when you go to
sleep. You should also sleep on a towel if you want to keep
the sheets and pillow dry.

How to Lose Weight after Giving Birth?

You will lose at least ten pounds of weight immediately
after you give birth and will lose a few more pounds in the
first week. It is a good idea to reach your ideal weight during
this time regardless of how much weight you may have gained
during your pregnancy. You should be active and consume a
healthy diet, which will help to boost your energy levels. You
will feel much better if you have enough energy. You will not
develop any health conditions, like high blood pressure and
diabetes, if you reach a healthy weight. If you want to have
another baby in the future, it is important that you reach
your ideal weight before your second pregnancy. Let us look
at some tips you can use to reach a healthy weight:

- Speak to your doctor about the weight you have gained and ask them to help you identify a way to reach your ideal weight.
- Limit your intake of processed foods and sweets.
- Follow a healthy diet.
- Drink a lot of water.
- Ask your doctor to help you understand how active you can be after you have given birth, especially if you have had a cesarean. Always begin slowly and increase the activity over time. You can swim or walk, but make sure that you stay active.
- You do burn a few calories when you breastfeed.
- Never try to lose too much weight because your body will need nutrients to heal. You will also reduce the supply of milk in your breasts if you lose weight too fast.
- You may not lose weight quickly, and this is fine. Do not be upset about it. Your body will take time to get back in shape. It is important that you stay fit for a longer time than worry about getting into shape immediately after you give birth.

What skin changes can happen after giving birth?

You will have some stretch marks on your abdomen and belly since you skin stretched when you were pregnant. Some women also have stretch marks on their bottom, thighs and hips. These stretch marks will not disappear after you give birth, but they will fade. You can apply different lotions or creams on your skin. That being said, these lotions and creams do not make these marks go away. They merely help to reduce the itching around those marks.

. . .

What hair changes can happen after giving birth?

You may have noticed that your hair was fuller and thicker during your pregnancy, and this is because the hormone levels in your body reduced hair loss. After you give birth, you will notice that your hair has started to thin out, and you may lose a lot of hair. You will stop losing hair after six months, and your hair will return to its normal volume in a year. If you want to avoid losing hair, you can do the following:

- Consume large quantities of fruit and vegetables. The nutrients will protect your hair and help it grow.
- Always be gentle with your hair. Do not wear braids, rollers or tight ponytails. These will stress your hair and pull it out.
- Always set your hair dryer to cool when you use it.

When do you get your period again after pregnancy?

Your period will start between the sixth and eighth week after you have given birth. This only happens when you are not breastfeeding. If you are feeding, your period will not start for a few months. Some women do not get their period until they stop feeding. If your period returns, it will not be the same as it was before your pregnancy. It could either be shorter or longer. It will soon return to how it used to be before your pregnancy.

When can you get pregnant again?

Doctors and physicians recommend that women give their body at least six weeks to heal after they give birth. This means that they can only have sex after six weeks. Even when your body is ready to have sex, you must be careful since you can get pregnant very easily. You will need to ovulate before you get your next period, and it will take your body at least six weeks before it can ovulate.

If you do not want to get pregnant again, you should use birth control, like intrauterine devices, pills, condoms and implants. Speak to your doctor or midwife about the birth control that you should use, especially if you are feeding. Some birth controls will reduce the supply of milk.

It is always a good idea to wait for at least eighteen months before you become pregnant again. When you increase the time between your pregnancies, you can reduce the risk of premature birth or low birth weight.

What Should You Do When You Feel Stressed Or Overwhelmed?

It is important for you to understand that your baby did not come with instructions. You will be overwhelmed and under a lot of stress when you are taking care of your baby. There is a lot that you will need to think about when it comes to a baby.

- Speak to your partner and let them know how you feel. Allow them to help you take care of the baby
- Ask your family and friends for help, and make sure that you let them know what it is exactly that you need them to do.
- Look for a support group with new mothers
- Always consume the right food, and make sure that you are always active
- Avoid consuming hard drugs, street drugs or

alcohol. These substances will make it harder for you to handle the stress.

What are baby blues and postpartum depression?

Women sometimes are upset or sad after they have given birth to a baby. This phenomenon is called postpartum blues or baby blues. You may feel this way a few days after you give birth, and this feeling can last up to three weeks. You do not have to treat this feeling since it goes away on its own.

Postpartum depression, on the other hand, is a state of depression that women go into once they have given birth to their baby. If you suffer from postpartum depression, you will have strong feelings of worry, anxiety, tiredness and sadness, and these feelings will last for a very long time after you give birth. You will find it difficult to take care of yourself and your baby if you suffer from this type of depression. You will need to get yourself checked and treated. This is one of the most common forms of depression that women face after they give birth.

#1 How to Deal With Baby Blues

- Try to sleep as much as you can
- Avoid any harmful drugs, street drugs and alcohol since these will affect your mood. There is a possibility that you may feel worse after you consume these substances.
- Ask your partner to help you. You can also reach out to family and friends. Let them know what you feel and tell them how they can help you.
- Spend some time outside the house.

- Meet with other mothers.
- If you are upset or have these feelings for more than two weeks, speak to your doctor or midwife.

#2 *How to Deal With Postpartum Depression*

- Speak to your doctor or midwife
- Understand what PPD is and what the risk factors are
- Learn more about the signs and symptoms
- Ask your doctor or midwife to help you understand how you can treat PPD

How can you handle going back to work or school?

It will definitely be hard for you to leave your baby at home all day with a family member, friend or a caregiver. It is also hard to trust the caregiver fully, and you and your partner may disagree on what is the best way to care for your child. You will be upset about the fact that you cannot stay at home with your baby. Let us see what you can do about this:

- Discuss how you want to care for your child with your partner. You should work on the finances and see how much you can spend. You should also talk to each other about the type of care you want to give your child. For instance, you can hire a caregiver who will come to your house and take care of the baby. Alternatively, you can drop your baby at a childcare center when you are away at work.
- You can ask family and friends to advise you on

childcare. You can either use the same service as them or ask them if you can use the same person.

- If you want to use a childcare center, make sure that you obtain all the information about the people working at the center. You should also call other parents who use the center to see what they think about the center.
- You should ask your boss if it is okay for you to slowly ease into work. You can work for a few hours from home at first, and then begin to work full time.

How can you and your partner get used to being new parents?

You and your partner are both getting used to having a third person in your house. Your partner is probably as nervous and stressed as you are, so make sure that you do not get irritated with them. Try to rely on each other and figure things out together. Let us look at what you both should do:

- Learn how to take care of your baby together. Take some baby-care classes or read some books to understand better.
- Do not try to do everything on your own. You should always talk to your partner and ask them to help with the baby.
- Learn to communicate. You should always talk about your feelings. This is the only way you can ensure that neither of you is frustrated.
- Always make time for each other. You can either go out for dinner or take a walk. Let someone take care of your baby for an hour.

- You should be open with your partner about sex, and make sure that you both are aware of when you can have sex again. If you do not want to speak directly to your partner about this, ask your doctor or midwife to speak to them.

CONCLUSION

Thank you for purchasing the book.

Pregnancy is a time of joy, but it is also a time when you will experience numerous changes in your body and in your life. It is important to learn how to deal with these changes. Over the course of the book, you will gather information about what causes stress during pregnancy and what you can do to overcome that stress, among other information.

I hope you have a calm and peaceful pregnancy and wish you luck on your journey.

SOURCES

https://www.womansday.com/health-fitness/womens-health/g2934/toxic-chemicals-to-avoid-when-pregnant/

https://www.babycentre.co.uk/a552044/11-ways-to-survive-stress-in-pregnancy

https://www.babycentre.co.uk/a547370/the-basics-of-good-sleep-in-pregnancy

https://www.self.com/story/8-important-things-women-forget-to-do-after-having-a-baby

https://www.marchofdimes.org/pregnancy/your-body-after-baby-the-first-6-weeks.aspx

CPSIA information can be obtained
at www.ICGtesting.com
Printed in the USA
BVHW040212290520
580541BV00015B/507